Bringing User Experience to Healthcare Improvement

The concepts, methods and practices of experience-based design

Paul Bate BA, PhD
Professor of Health Services Management
Royal Free & University College Medical School
University College London

and

Glenn Robert BA, MSc, PhD
Principal Research Fellow
Royal Free & University College Medical School
University College London

Foreword by

Lynne Maher
Head of Innovation Practice
NHS Institute for Innovation and Improvement

Radcliffe Publishing
Oxford • New York

Radcliffe Publishing Ltd
18 Marcham Road
Abingdon
Oxon OX14 1AA
United Kingdom

www.radcliffe-oxford.com
Electronic catalogue and worldwide online ordering facility.

British Library Cataloguing in Publication Data

A catalogue record for this book is available from the British Library.

ISBN-13: 978 1 84619 176 3

Typeset by Lapiz Digital Services, Chennai, India
Printed and bound by TJ International Ltd, Padstow, Cornwall, UK

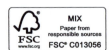

MIX
Paper from
responsible sources
FSC® C013056

We had a big incident at the hospital. Various things had gone wrong. It was the day after that they said he was going to die. And we had a fantastic nurse on the High Dependency Unit for most of the day and I'd heard a lovely doctor say to the nurse, 'Look, go between glucose and saline.' She said, 'I won't chart it because I know, if it goes below 10, give him glucose, and if it's above 10, give him saline. I'll just leave that,' and she went, 'That's fine.' Consequently, what happened though, glucose wasn't charted on there. J's sugar dropped to four, that nurse had gone off and he was on an insulin drip, and I said, 'Can we put the glucose drip up?' And they said, 'No. No, it's got to be saline because glucose isn't charted.' And like, 'He's diabetic. He will go into a coma. You're giving him insulin and he's four, and it's just because . . .' And they said, 'It's not charted. Legally, we're bound.' And the nurse brought the doctor around and the doctor said, 'I support what the nurse said.' And then went. He didn't even stop to say, 'What's his history?' or to find out what's going on. Again, I think they found me a very difficult person to have on the ward because, you know, I would question them. Anyway, I thought the best bet is to burst into tears, but I was so frustrated like, why can't they understand this? It's four. His blood sugar is four. He needs to have glucose. 'Please can you ring the nurse who was on here before? Just ring her up.' 'No, we don't call nurses at home.' 'Okay, I can understand that. However, what are we going to do? Are we going to wait until she comes in next morning and then find that he's dropped into a coma?' And then she did call the doctor at home, because I said 'The doctor said I could call her any time, so can you please do that and just check.' She was fantastic. And the following morning, the Sister called me in and she said, 'Look, how can we avoid this happening again?'

Contents

Foreword

Can you imagine what it would be like if we moved from a health service that does things for its patients to one that is patient-led? Where patients and staff together have specifically designed the service so that it provides the best experience that you could hope for? This compelling book illustrates a new approach to redesigning health systems so that they truly meet the needs of patients and staff, the very people who are experiencing them. If you are a healthcare professional – indeed anyone who wants to be involved in making health services better for patients, their families and carers – by picking up this book you have taken the first step in what I believe could be one of the most exciting and rewarding journeys of your professional life.

In their preface, the authors Paul and Glenn talk about an 'expedition' and a 'white-water ride'. This metaphor also reflects the journey that unfolded for a small team who were brought together by the NHS Institute for Innovation and Improvement to specifically develop and test new methods of enabling patients to participate as equals in improving healthcare services. The team included patients, family members, healthcare staff, healthcare improvers, researchers and designers. Together they moved from understanding the initial concepts of 'user centric design' and 'co-designing for user experience', through to designing the methods used to draw these concepts together, before testing this new approach to improving experiences of healthcare, and finally, illustrating the profound effect and practical impact that experience-based design (EBD) brings.

The approach demonstrates how a combination of existing and new techniques can be used together. For example, the well-established NHS practice of 'process mapping' (analysing the chronological steps in the patient process) can be enhanced by 'experience or emotional mapping'. Here, service users and families create maps that illustrate their journey as they have felt it. They do not focus on every step but rather the critical points where they are profoundly touched by the service, leading to a positive or negative experience. Gathering stories or narratives have been combined with picture diaries or video film, which has brought to life the nuances that impact massively on the service provided and received. Project teams have been established but with equal partnership between patients and staff who have successfully developed and implemented changes to improve the delivery and experience of care.

The combination of a robust research approach, incorporating design methods and, critically, expertise from both patients and staff, demonstrates the true value of effectively achieving 'research into practice'. The significance of this synergy should not be underestimated and will be appreciated by researchers, front line professionals and patients alike.

The NHS system reform programme, set out in *Creating a Patient-Led NHS*, represents a profound change in the ways we need to think about, organise and deliver NHS services. Experience-based design will fundamentally change the relationships in the system, between patients and care-givers, between commissioners and providers of care, redefining the way that NHS Services are delivered. Whether you are a chief executive, nurse, health strategist, porter, radiographer, doctor, in fact anyone working in health services, the core question you should ask is, 'How can we design services that are as much about how patients feel, and about their whole experience of care, as they are about functionality and good processes?' Experience-based design must become the core principle that you use when delivering health services, recognising patients, carers and families as producers and participants rather than just receivers of healthcare services. You need to enable users to play a much greater role in identifying needs, proposing solutions, testing them out and implementing them jointly with care providers.

How many of us, when we think about patient involvement, automatically think about patient surveys, forums, user-groups and all the other valuable but nevertheless standard ways of demonstrating that we are listening to our patients? And what do we do once we've heard them? Undoubtedly, we walk away with more resolve to make things better, often with personal actions to be undertaken with staff, but rarely with a process in mind or resource to help achieve important improvements. If I had to share just one thing with readers of this book it would be this – experience-based design isn't just a totally achievable way of engaging with patients to find out what they think about the services we provide; it is a systematic process that we can follow, it is a true combination of human resources, it's about inviting patients themselves to work alongside us to make those changes happen. It is clear that patients, carers and families want to help, we need to let them.

However readers use this book, and whatever they take away from it, one thing is certain – it will be hard for anyone to see patients and service users in quite the same light again. So often, as skilled and experienced professionals, we think we know what patients need and want – asking them is sometimes a courtesy. Experience-based design is powerful – it dares us to go deeper and provides a new dialogue and dynamic with patients and their carers. The design and delivery of healthcare services cannot stay the same once this happens.

Dr Lynne Maher
Head of Innovation Practice
NHS Institute for Innovation and Improvement
April 2007

Preface and acknowledgements

The origins of this book lie in our close collaboration over the past five and more years with patients and carers and those leading the modernisation and change agenda within the English National Health Service (NHS). Viewed as a journey this can only be described as something of a white-water ride in terms of the excitement, stimulation, and frequently knuckle-biting experiences, it has given to us all. This is not surprising given the scale and complexity of the 10-year improvement plan in the NHS. Beginning in July 2000 it was that plan which brought users, practitioners and academics together in the first place, with the sheer and uncompromising ambition contained in its vision to 'transform' the NHS and bring about a 'quality revolution' in the healthcare services it provides.

The plan has been described as 'the largest concerted systematic improvement effort ever undertaken, anywhere, in any industry'.[1] It is unsurprising, then, that the conventional organisation and change theories of us, the academics, and the established policies and practices of them, the practitioners, have been put to the severest of tests in this context – and sometimes found wanting. In some cases, this has meant that these theories and practices have had to be reshaped and remodelled; in other cases simply discarded as ineffective or unfit for purpose. Part of the journey itself – and very reminiscent of those of the early explorers – has involved the search for new conceptual and practice terrains, and new strains or species of theory or approach that might be better suited to the job in hand.

This book is the story of one such recent expedition which began in 2004 and initially took members of – what was then – the NHS Modernisation Agency and ourselves into the field of design and the design sciences. We went there to see whether there were any frameworks and methods being used in areas such as architecture and software computing that might have value in addressing some of the organisational design and development challenges facing the NHS. We are happy to say that this has generally proved to be the case and that our joint work in exploring and mining the rich territory of design is continuing apace. However, it is not this story we shall specifically be relating here.

While emerging from this bigger journey to the New World (for organisation and service designers at least) of design and the design sciences, this book is, rather, more of a trip up one of its narrower creeks or tributaries, one that we all stumbled upon almost by chance as we tacked back and forth on our travels. On the maps you will find many different names for the particular location in question, 'participatory', 'user-based' or 'interactive' design being the most popular. In the end, however, we settled on a less well-known title for this book: 'experience-based design' (EBD). We did this, first, because, while EBD does involve user participation in the design process (a point we later make explicit by adding the prefix 'co-' to make it co-design), it is narrower in focus, being a particular form of user involvement that uniquely focuses upon the concept of designing for the human experience; second, because it makes useful and immediate connections with an already well-established healthcare discourse on 'the patient experience'; and, third, because there is a pressing problem that remains to be addressed in health-care, namely that that same discourse has become so familiar, so much part of everyday values and NHS talk, that we rarely stop to think what 'experience' is, and therefore are in danger of missing why it is so important to service design.

We want to take readers back up this particular design tributary at a relatively leisurely pace in the hope that during the journey they may find things of inter-est to take back and adapt for use in their own work environment. However, the structure of the book recognises that each will have their own particular interests and preferences that they wish to pursue. The book is organised into three parts – concepts, methods and practices – so that, after a brief introductory chapter that sets the context for what follows, readers may turn immediately to the pages of most interest to them. For example, healthcare practitioners and improvement specialists may find it helpful to 'begin at the back' with the final part (practices), which has a detailed description of a case study of an EBD approach as applied to a head and neck cancer service, before looping back as necessary through meth-ods and then into the first part on concepts.

One warning: in this book readers will hopefully find balance in our arguments and close scrutiny of the evidence, but they will not find neutrality or detach-ment. We are passionate about seeing much greater patient participation in serv-ice design and a much greater focus upon designing better experiences for them, not just better processes. But we are also frustrated: customers *are* increasingly becoming part of the service and experience creation process in organisations generally, and our question is why healthcare seems to be dragging its heels. With this book, at least, we hope that ignorance of the topic will not be the cause.

Since time began travellers and explorers have needed their expedition spon-sors. Our generous sponsor for the bigger 'Design' expedition was the NHS Modernisation Agency, while the case-study work described in Chapter 9 was funded by the Agency's successor organisation, the NHS Institute for Innovation and Improvement (NHS III). We are particularly grateful to Helen Bevan, Director of Service Transformation at the NHS III, for her energetic support and deeply insightful contributions to this topic since our search began, and, no less, her constant insistence upon 'relevance' and value for money for the NHS. As we write, readers may like to know that an EBD toolkit is in development – led by the NHS III – and may now be available since we went to press. Helen is a true pioneer in the improvement field and a fantastic travelling companion. We also thank those who related their – often deeply moving – stories to us and from which we have cited extracts, including David Shiers and Jo Norton of the National Early Intervention Programme of NIMHE (National Institute for Mental Health in England) and Rethink, and Barbara Monroe, Chief Executive of St. Christopher's Hospice. We would also like to thank our fellow colleagues and team members from the EBD case study described in Chapter 9 of this book, namely Elaine Hide and Kate Jones, Deborah Szebeko and Ivo Gormley, John Pickles and Carole Glover (both of whom managed to play a major role in the project while maintaining a full clinical workload), and Lynne Maher (Head of Innovation Practice, NHS III) who so effectively took over the helm from Helen as we moved into rougher seas of piloting, testing and disseminating EBD as a new way of approaching change in the NHS. We are particularly grateful to Elaine, Deborah and Ivo for their contributions to Chapter 9. We would especially like to thank Elaine, who led the work locally and collated some of the material on which Chapter 10 draws. Most importantly, we acknowledge the invaluable contributions of the head and neck cancer patients and carers themselves who gave so freely of their time and energy over a 12-month period of their lives filled with many other competing demands and obvious stresses. It is their experiences we describe, and without which this book would not have been possible – experiences that were always so willingly and generously shared, even by some who were in the final stages of their life.

The broad suggestion that the design sciences might have much to offer those leading change in an organisational context, building on the initial work of organisational theorists like Joan van Aken and George Romme, is one in which we have become increasingly interested, indeed convinced by. For readers intrigued – like us – by this wider proposition we suggest they also turn to a special edition of the *Journal of Applied Behavioral Science* to be published in 2007, which was guest-edited by one of the authors of this book (PB) and has several contributions by NHS staff and associates. In this context we would like to thank Jean Bartunek (Boston College), Dick Woodman (Texas A & M University), Michael Manning (New Mexico State University), Marcel Veenswijk (Free University of Amsterdam) and all the authors (many writing from a healthcare perspective) who contributed papers to the special edition and the accompanying American Academy of Management 'showcase' symposium in 2006 for their encouragement and support in this venture.

We are grateful to the publishers of the journal *Quality and Safety in Health Care* for granting permission to reproduce extracts (including Figures 1.1 and 1.2) from an overview paper we had previously written on this topic. The description of the case study presented in Chapter 9 draws in part on a paper that will appear in the special edition of the *Journal of Applied Behavioral Science* in 2007. Again, we are grateful to the publishers for permission to reprint extracts (including Figures 9.1, 9.2 and 9.3) from the paper here. Figure 2.4 is reproduced by permission of Peter Morville, Semantics Studios; Figure 8.1 by permission of Matrix Research & Consultancy; Figure 10.1 by permission of the Health Care Commission; Figure 11.1 by permission of The MIT Press; and Figure 11.2 by permission of the MIT Sloan School of Management. Our design partners in the case study described in Chapter 9 – *thinkpublic* – provided Figures 9.1, 9.5 and D1 and prepared the tools used in the various patient, staff and co-design events described in Chapter 9. Finally, we thank the reviewers of our earlier papers on this subject for their comments and suggestions, many of which have manifested themselves in improvements to this book.

Paul Bate and Glenn Robert
April 2007

Reference

1 Berwick D, Institute for Healthcare Improvement. As cited in: Greenhalgh T, Robert G, Bate SP *et al. Diffusion of Innovations in Health Service Organisations. A Systematic Literature Review.* Oxford: Blackwell; 2005. p. 25.

About the authors

Paul Bate holds the Chair of Health Services Management within the Medical School, University College London. A social anthropologist and organisation theorist by background, Paul works with clinicians, senior managers, and staff at all levels of the NHS to help bring about major improvements in health services. He is the author of four books and numerous journal articles on quality, service development and change, many of these with co-author Glenn Robert.

Glenn Robert is Principal Research Fellow within the Medical School, University College London. A sociologist by background, Glenn's research centres on quality and service improvement in healthcare, with a focus on the policy implementation process at the local level and securing sustained change within healthcare organisations. His latest book with his co-author Paul Bate and others (Greenhalgh T *et al.* (2005) *Diffusion of Innovations in Health Service Organisations*) was the 2006 winner of the Baxter Award for the most outstanding contribution to healthcare management in Europe.

Glossary

A&E	Accident & Emergency
CBPR	community-based participatory research
DI	Discovery Interview
EBD	experience-based co-design
ED	experience design
HCI	human–computer interaction
HDU	high dependency unit
HICSS	Hawaii International Conference on Systems Sciences
ICAS	independent complaints advocacy service
ICU	intensive care unit
MDT	multi-disciplinary team
MSC	most significant change
MUDs	multiple user dimensions
NAO	National Audit Office
NHS	National Health Service
NHS III	National Health Service Institute for Innovation and Improvement
NIMHE	National Institute for Mental Health in England
OD	organisational development
OS	organisational studies
PALS	patient advice and liaison services
PAT	'Patients as Teachers' programme
PCD	people-centred design
PD	participatory design
PEG	percutaneous endoscopic gastrostomy
PPI	Patient and Public Involvement
PSA	public service agreement
SIGs	special interest groups
TQM	total quality management
UCD	user-centric design
UK	United Kingdom
US	United States
USP	unique selling point
UX or UXD	user experience design

Chapter 1

Introduction: bringing the user experience to healthcare

Experiences are one of the most valuable memories we have . . . Successful experiences are valuable both financially and emotionally and the more we learn about how to create them (whether through approach, process, understanding, or specific criteria), the better the experiences we can create and the more enriching our lives can become. (Nathan Shedroff)

Service users as 'quality detectives'

For many years the best service organisations in the private sector have been aware of the need to manage the 'customer service experience' with the same rigour as they bring to their functional and operational components. Rather than regarding their customers as the passive recipients of their service, they see them as 'detectives',[1] actively sniffing out 'experience clues' concerning what they are being offered in terms of the reliability and technical quality of the service (cognitive functional clues), the appearance and presentation of the service (emotional, sensory and aesthetic clues), and the interactive quality of the service (behavioural and linguistic clues). As they engage with the service, customers and users are very much in 'smart detective' mode, and it is on the strength of these clues that they 'rate' and judge their overall experience, and make calculations as to whether to stay with or switch to new providers in future.

> *Whether managers put it all together – or don't – customers do. They work out the 'clue math.' They add up the clues and compute intricate and unconscious calculations that . . . shape their assessment of the service's quality.*[1]

We hear with increasing, almost tedious, regularity of the lengths to which the leading service organisations like Starbucks, Federal Express, IBM, Xerox, HP (Hewlett-Packard), the Ritz Carlton, Hilton or Marriott Hotels, and Southwest Airlines[2] are prepared to go in order to make the customer's experience a good – nay, excellent – one, the simple logic being that a good customer experience is good customer service; the experience is the service. Many, like the Hampton Inn, have also been at pains to 'put their money where their mouth is', in this case offering an unconditional service guarantee that if guests encounter any kind of service failure during their stay – a plumbing, air conditioning, or noise problem, for example – then they can stay the night free.

The United Kingdom (UK) National Health Service (NHS), or for that matter any other healthcare system, is clearly not the Hampton Inn but it does have all of the features of a service organisation, and is facing similar, if not much greater, pressures to become more user-centred. To this extent, we shall argue that it is no different from any other service organisation with regard to the central importance of the 'customer experience', and the fact that this should be the guide in everything that it thinks and does as an organisation. And while the NHS may sometimes mistake horizontal patients for passive patients, it can rest assured that it will find the same expert detectives and sleuths as may be found in any other service or customer setting. Indeed, Berry and colleagues suggest that in a hospital setting, for obvious reasons, patients can be expected to come especially high on the 'smart detective scale':

> *The more important, variable, complex and personal the service, the more detective work customers are likely to do as they sense experience clues. Hospital patients, for example, can be expected to be quite detective-like if they are alert. Few service experiences are more important, variable, complex, and personal than being hospitalised, and patients are likely to be eager for any evidence of the hospital's competence and caring.*[1]

One healthcare system that *has* apparently passed the smart detective test with flying colours is the Mayo Clinic in Rochester and Scottsdale in the United States (US).[3] The secret in their case was to be patient-centred even down to the smallest visual and experiential clues and to strictly follow the creed: 'Understand the story you want to tell, and then make sure your people and your facilities provide evidence of that story to customers, day in and day out.'

Today, designers in all walks of life – not just service designers but product designers and organisational designers in the private sector,[4] too – are waking up to the importance of placing the 'user experience' at the heart of the design process. However, because it is the profit motive that is usually driving such an interest (i.e. good user experience is good for business), we are only too aware that healthcare organisations, and especially those in the public sector, might easily choose to exempt themselves from this wider movement, or at least choose to pursue it with less vigour. They would be wrong to do this, we believe, for just as private organisations have become exposed to growing market choice, in which a coffee-shop customer who is dissatisfied with any aspect of his or her experience can – and often does – switch his or her loyalties elsewhere to any one of a plethora of other providers, so too are healthcare organisations beginning to wake up to the implications of wider patient choice. There is a growing possibility that disgruntled patients may also choose to 'take their coffee' elsewhere.

However, economic pragmatism is obviously not the only – or even primary – reason why healthcare needs to be considering a more conscious and committed move towards the notion of user-centric service design. In some ways, humanistic and cultural considerations are far more important, especially in a context where people are obviously not there for pleasure or enjoyment but for essential, sometimes life or death, clinical reasons. The experience design movement says it is no longer sufficient to seek to *meet* users' expectations but to *exceed* them in situations like these. This is a mindset which, though possibly alien to healthcare institutions in the past, must be the right one for the stressful situations in which patients and carers find themselves, and absolutely in accord with the culture of 'continuous improvement' that many 'modernising' healthcare systems have been striving towards over the last five to ten years, including the NHS. Thus, whereas in the past, people may have pointed to the high satisfaction ratings given by patients following treatment as sufficient reason for not seeking to further improve the patient experience (which as we shall argue later can lead to terrible self-deception and complacency on the part of the providers) it is now becoming widely accepted that this cannot be defended given that the baseline expectation was often quite low in the first place.

At this early point of our argument, and at the slight risk of taking away some of the seriousness surrounding this issue, we would remind readers of the 'happy slave syndrome' found in psychology which relates the apocryphal story of eighteenth-century slaves who, when being handed a satisfaction questionnaire, rated their lot as 5 out of 5 every time (5 being most satisfied), (a) because they were simply relieved to be alive not dead, and (b) because they had only been beaten by their masters three times that week not the five of the previous week. This is the issue of regressive expectations, the irony of the story being that the lower the expectation, say of a health service, the more 'satisfied' one is likely to be with it (and, equally, the higher the expectation, the greater the likelihood of disappointment or dissatisfaction). We will return to the difference between satisfaction and experience in Chapter 10 but alert the reader to it now: for us (and others[5]) the difference is far more than a semantic one and has important implications for the way in which healthcare services develop and improve.

What is there left to learn about designing better healthcare systems?

Against the backcloth of recent healthcare reform in England, we note that there is a growing recognition that while the process and current pace of change will continue, the way in which that change happens will need to be different in the next five years from what has been happening during the last five years, especially with regard to present levels of patient-centredness and involvement. For example, the recent NHS Operating Framework for 2006–7 confirms a change from 'targets-driven' to 'incentives-driven' change, expressing it thus:

> . . . *[a commitment to] reform the health system fundamentally, so that change is driven more by incentives to* **respond to patients** *than by top-down target setting . . . old methods of top-down performance management will not be sufficient to deliver this.*[6] (emphasis added)

Internationally, too, there is an awareness that existing healthcare systems and processes in their present form are not going to deliver all of what is required for the future. For instance, a survey of almost 7,000 patients from six countries found – in all of the countries – significant numbers reporting safety risks, poor care co-ordination and deficiencies in care for chronic conditions.[7] The countries in this 2005 telephone survey were Australia, Canada, Germany, New Zealand, the UK and the US. More than one in four patients in each country (28% to 32%) said risks were not completely explained during their hospital stay. In all countries, sizeable majorities of patients said doctors had not always reviewed all their medications during the past year, and one-third or more reported infrequent reviews. Across the countries, one-sixth to one-quarter of patients said doctors only sometimes, rarely, or never made goals of care and treatment clear or gave them clear instructions. In terms of errors (defined as a medical mistake, medication error or test error in the past two years) 34% of US respondents reported at least one error. The lowest figure (22%) was reported by respondents from the UK.

In attempting to improve the quality of healthcare, governments around the world are engaged in intensive efforts to bring about radical and sustainable changes in their health services through various programmatic – and, despite the rhetoric, still largely top-down – approaches to improvement and effectiveness.[8] Driving these efforts is the perceived shortfall between what is currently being provided and what people need, want and (should) expect by way of access to safe, high-quality healthcare. For instance, McGlynn and colleagues report on the mediocre state of quality of healthcare in the US.[9] Looking across 439 quality indicators for 30 acute and chronic conditions, the authors document that only 54.9% of patients receive recommended care; in other words 45.1% did not – an astounding finding. Few would dispute that this figure is probably the same for many other countries including the UK. The Institute of Medicine, in its seminal 2001 report *Crossing the Quality Chasm: A New Health System for the 21st Century*, describes the 'chasm' between the unacceptably poor standards of current care delivery systems and what it could and should be in the context of the US.[10] It provides a challenging manifesto for transformation of the American healthcare system as a whole. Similarly, the Australian Council for Safety and Quality in Health Care has set out a radical platform for investment in health systems redesign, system capacity building, cultural development and enabling patients to be partners in their own care.[11]

The starting point for our argument is, therefore, that existing perspectives, methods and approaches to improvement, and the underlying theories that drive them, can not be relied upon to deliver the required change in the time and on the scale required;[8] hence the need to widen and intensify the search for 'better' and more effective theories and approaches to large-scale change and whole systems transformation. To this end the (recently dissolved) NHS Modernisation Agency had already begun to investigate many new territories, including models of design. However, while there is now broad acceptance of the need for new and innovative approaches to innovation and service transformation – a key role for the Modernisation Agency's successor organisation, the NHS Institute for Innovation and Improvement (NHS III),[12] and the Patient and Public Involvement (PPI) resource centre (which began work in January 2006) – most sources are still less than clear about what these approaches are, or where they will come from.

The three elements of good design

As far as healthcare is concerned, one rich, and as yet largely untapped, corpus of knowledge and ideas is the wider field of design sciences and the design professions, such as architecture, computer, product and graphic design. The question we pose in this regard is: what can we learn from the design professions about how to design better healthcare systems? The relevance of such a link is that 'good design' of healthcare services, we would argue, is essentially no different from good design in any sphere, be it a product or service,[13] this being a function of three things (*see* Figure 1.1).

An exercise we often run when discussing the design sciences with groups of healthcare managers and practitioners is to ask them to think about some of the great 'icons' of design (Concorde, the Eiffel Tower, a Bialetti coffee maker and an Apple computer are favourite examples or hotels or airlines that provide

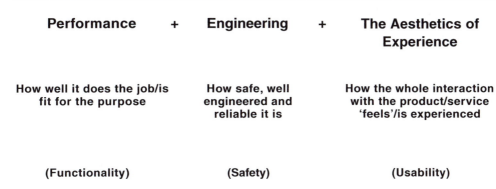

Performance	+	Engineering	+	The Aesthetics of Experience
How well it does the job/is fit for the purpose		How safe, well engineered and reliable it is		How the whole interaction with the product/service 'feels'/is experienced
(Functionality)		(Safety)		(Usability)

Figure 1.1   The three elements of good design. *Source*: Berkun.[14]

exemplary five-star service), and ask themselves: 'What is it that marks out these products and services as being so great?' What often comes as a surprise is their discovery that, despite the huge differences between these icons in both scale and substance, the underlying reason they are so great is that they all score highly on the three basic elements in Figure 1.1. In other words, they are great because they not only 'do the job' with ruthless efficiency, but are safe and reliable, and feel great to interact with or use (the issue of interactivity and usability). These three magic ingredients of great design have been best articulated by the designer Scott Berkun, who uses the example of the Brooklyn Bridge, and John Roebling (its designer), to express this 'noble idea' of design as aesthetics + engineering + performance:

> *It had to be beautiful, reliable and functional. They saw their role not just to build something that would transport people, or last 50 years or 200, but to contribute to the landscape and the human experience of everyone that came into contact with their creation. Every sketch and diagram John Roebling made considered not only its physical purpose and structure, but also its visual appearance to those walking on the bridge, and those looking at it from across the river.*[14]

This sentiment reminds us of the power of design to deal not only with the purpose but also the spirit of a thing. As Lewis Mumford (cited by Berkun) once reflected:

> *It is the spirit behind the Brooklyn Bridge, and the spirit in the structure itself, the spirit that you anticipate and appreciate even if you've never studied engineering, even if you've never studied aesthetics. It's there. And in one degree or another people that use it and have their eyes open respond to it.*[14]

Few healthcare practitioners would probably disagree with the idea that 'spirit' is just as important in healthcare, if not more so.

We put these two quotations up front deliberately to provoke readers to reflect on whether there still is or needs to be a similar noble idea in modern healthcare that acts as the North Star for design in all spheres of its activity. A health service may be a far cry from an American bridge but perhaps the idea of contributing to 'the landscape and the human experience of everyone' is not that far off the mark as an equally admirable health aim and ideal. In just such a vein,

Sophie Petit-Zeman describes a book she wrote about the contemporary NHS as being:

> ... about clawing back tender, loving health care, giving and receiving it, before we lose sight of what it is. It's about finding a way to restore the NHS to what it's there for, to rein in its spiralling complexity, before it's too late. Bringing the health care debate back to where it belongs, it [the book] sets out reasons why getting better is about people, not about politics, professional posturing and pride. Well or ill, we're in it, together.[15]

One aspect of the design approach that healthcare practitioners might therefore find attractive is the suggestion that, while today's engineers (including business process re-engineers) deal mainly with performance and reliability, it is only the 'designers' who put spirit and aesthetics back into the equation. Below we expand upon each of the three elements from Figure 1.1.

Performance or functionality supports the core of any service because it addresses the problem that brings the customer or user to that organisation in the first place. Customers come for solutions and will judge the organisation on how far it provides them. This means that nothing trumps performing the service right the first time.[1] On the other hand, a core failure in this element, for example a course of treatment that does not work out as expected, is likely to provoke a stronger negative reaction than the other two elements combined. In an award-winning study on why customers leave one service supplier for another, Keaveney found that 44% of the sample switched because of a core service failure; core service failure was the most frequently mentioned reason for switching.[16] Many NHS patients may not yet have the same luxury or ease of switching hospitals as, say, between coffee shops on the high street[17] but it is certainly true that a perception of a badly performed core service (for example, a botched hip replacement operation) is the strongest reason why they do not want to return to the same surgeon or hospital.

Reliability and engineering are about how safe and dependable the service is or is felt to be ('the ability to perform the promised service dependably and accurately'). For example, in a series of studies across 13 different services, customers rated reliability (planes, trains, equipment, system and processes not breaking down) as the most important dimension in meeting their expectations in every case.[18] Similar or higher importance ratings might be expected in high-risk hospital situations where even a simple mix-up in a procedure can lead to injury or death. Just to give a sense of the scale of 'safety incidents' in healthcare, in 2003–4 there were 885,832 patient safety incidents and near misses in the NHS.[19] A follow-up survey found that in 2004–5 there were around 974,000 reported incidents and near misses. Hospital-acquired infections may increase these figures by around 300,000 incidents (around 30% of which may have been preventable). The most common incidents reported were patient injury (due to falls), followed by medication errors, equipment-related incidents, record documentation error and communication failure. An analysis of hospital surveys in the same report found that in 2004–5 there were some 2,181 deaths because of recorded patient safety incidents but it is acknowledged that there is significant under-reporting of deaths and serious incidents. Other published estimates of death as a result of patient safety incidents range from 840 to 34,000 per annum but in reality the NHS simply does not know. Whatever the actual state of affairs may be, these figures show that the NHS still has a considerable way to go with regard to this second aspect of good design, particularly in comparison to other service organisations such as the airlines.

Aesthetics may appear to be the softer cousin next to the other two elements – and perhaps viewed by some as the icing on the cake. They should not be deluded. This third design element covers a huge spectrum, ranging from 'hard' technological and scientific issues about 'utility', 'usability', 'interactivity', and the 'user-interface',[20–22] as in how a driver interacts with the car or radiographer with the X-ray machine (or as Gadney[23] puts it – rather more prosaically – 'fumbling helplessly while trying to open a compact disc or a packet of ham has become a daily headache of modern life') to the aesthetic and artistic issues about 'appeal' and attraction (the emotional aspects of user experience[24]), and how it 'feels' to interact with these machines – or, for that matter, a service. We will bring out the range, differences and boundaries of the definition as we go on, not forgetting our broad argument that healthcare and healthcare design have engaged to a far lesser extent with this particular element. However, a point that needs to be made from the outset is that there is nothing fluffy or soft about this third aspect, or that it is simply the optional extra to the other two; it can also involve 'hard' life-or-death issues on a par with the other two elements. For example, how 'user-friendly' the interaction is between, say, the user and his or her car dashboard, X-ray machine, or blood analysis machine can make the difference between life and death.[25] Something that is more 'usable' is more likely to lead to fewer errors as well as leading to better performance, hence its strong link to the first two aspects of engineering and performance as well. For example, usability design has saved many lives through in-built 'forcing functions' to prevent errors:

> *A forcing function makes the user do something that prevents (or makes unlikely) some type of mistake. Many cars, for example, will not let you take the key out of the ignition unless the car is in a correct gear. This makes it very unlikely that you will leave the car in neutral when you leave your car, only to watch it slip down the hill and into your mother-in-law's new Lexus.*[26]

Similarly, many cars will not let you start them unless the gearstick is in 'park' position. Healthcare designers need to take urgent heed of this interactivity or usability factor, which not only applies to pieces of technology but also to processes. 'Clumsiness' in the care process, invariably a symptom of poor levels of usability and interactivity, will, for example, result in higher risk to patients at handovers between shifts or departments.

On the other hand, the importance of the 'softer' end of this element is that whereas functionality and engineering are usually most important in *meeting* customers' service expectations, aesthetic clues are most important in *exceeding* customers' expectations; hence they usually offer the richest potential for improving the quality of the service in terms of experience. This is the element where even the smallest things – a smile, a squeeze of the hand – can transform an 'acceptable' service experience into a 'superlative' one.

In its own way, healthcare has always been quite deeply involved with the first two elements of design: 'performance' in terms of the use of evidence-based practice, pathways and process design to ensure the clinical intervention is right; and 'engineering' in terms of clinical governance and standards to make it safer and more reliable (although making it *feel* safe may be a different matter). Petit-Zeman[15] uses the example of how patients used to die during operations because they were given nitrous oxide instead of oxygen but that this rarely happens now because you can no longer fit the oxygen tube on the nitrogen cylinder; the potential for error and harm has to all intents been 'designed out' (although, as the same author also points out, the technician who 'went at a cylinder with a hammer so he could put the tubes on the wrong way round' takes us back to well-intentioned humans – as in this example – messing things up even if systems are designed to stop them). But arguably healthcare has never engaged explicitly or to anything like the same extent with the third element – designing human experiences (as distinct from designing processes). For example, 'experience' barely receives a mention in the recent *Creating a Patient-Led NHS*[27] which suggests a more traditional mindset that continues to focus upon 'preference and choice', 'listening, understanding and responding', 'support, consultation and complaints', where patient influence rather than experience is the focus.

On the face of it, all this may sound – indeed may be – a little unfair in seeming to discount the huge amount of effort that has gone into putting the 'patient experience' at the top of the current political agenda, and making it a priority in recent Department of Health and other government policy documents. For example, 'Improve the patient and user experience' is one of four highly influential public service agreement (PSA) targets signed up to by the Department of Health from 2004 onwards,[28] which made a formal commitment to 'secure national improvements in NHS patient experience by 2008' (*see* page 167 for more details). Commitment is not the issue here, however, but what that means and how it is measured. The above phrase continues 'as measured by independently validated surveys', which reveals a concern we investigate later that it is patient attitudes and satisfaction – not experience – that is being measured (with all the problems associated with the 'happy slave syndrome' already mentioned). The final phrase, 'ensuring that individuals are fully involved in decisions about their health care, including choice of provider', also leaves us wondering whether the government is as clear as it should be as to the meaning and significance of 'experience'. Clearly choice and participation may be important ingredients of patient experience but it is also quite possible for patients to have lots of choice and participation yet still end up having a poor service experience. (Indeed our later case study shows that the patient experience may be worsened as the result of the patient being offered choice and participation on matters where he or she does not feel qualified to choose or participate.) The danger here is that the dogma of 'choice' and 'participation' may have ended up limiting the definition of 'experience' and underestimating the significance and potential of what might really be achieved under this banner. In this respect we believe the Secretary of State for Health may therefore have got it right when she invited the NHS to ask, 'How can we make our patients' and users' experiences better? How would it feel if it was me or my elderly mum?' In some ways these two questions frame the main aims of this book and EBD itself.

A wider trend

Patient involvement in healthcare design is part of a wider trend towards more 'bottom-up' public participation in organisational and social affairs. Witness, for example, the growing popularity of community-based participatory research (CBPR), which involves citizens and consumers both researching and designing services in health, education, local government and community development projects.[29-32] (*See* page 31 for further discussion of 'participation' as a key feature of the EBD approach.) For example, in England the Design Council's RED unit has advocated a 'co-creation' approach to health services.[33] The unit is testing such an approach in two projects: one focusing on a deprived community in the south-east of England and a second, in the north-west, working with patients and healthcare professionals to develop a new way of managing diabetes. The report on the first nine months of the two projects describes the work as:

> *part of a wider movement towards open welfare, in which the traditional distinction between producer and consumer – or in the welfare field between the public services and the client or patient – is transformed into networks of self-acting citizens, with flexible degrees of involvement, supported in a range of ways by professionals. In other words, the user becomes a producer, and as such needs skills, tools, information, means of communication and technical support.*[34]

This unit argues 'for a new approach which we call co-creation since a new set of relationships between users, workers and professionals lies at its heart'.

Experience-based design

Although still a distant horizon in healthcare, experience-based design (EBD), the subject of our book, might be regarded as an extension of the current NHS trajectory and part of this wider trend, and fortunately, therefore, does not, in our view, require starting anything from scratch. EBD is a user- (in this case patient- and carer-) focused design process with the goal of making user experience accessible to the designers, to allow them to conceive of designing experiences rather than designing services.[35,36] Experience is designated as 'how well people understand it, how they feel about it while they are using it, how well it serves its purpose, and how well it fits into the context in which they are using it'.[37] By identifying the main areas (or 'touch points') where people come into contact with the service and where their subjective experience is shaped, and therefore where the desired emotional and sensory connection needs to be established – and working with the front-line people who bring alive those various touch points – one can begin to design human experiences rather than just systems or processes.

On the present 'continuum of patient influence', starting from 'complaining' and 'information giving', to 'listening and responding', through to 'consulting/advising' – all of which are currently to be found within the NHS – EBD is one step on, being about equal partnership and the co-design of services.[13] Here, the traditional view of the user as a passive recipient of a product or service therefore gives way to the view of users as the co-designers of that product or service, as they join and become integrally bound up in the whole improvement and innovation process (*see* Figure 1.2).

There are obvious resonances here with the current, and much trumpeted, concept of 'patient-led services', but the 'co' in co-design is a significant and powerful

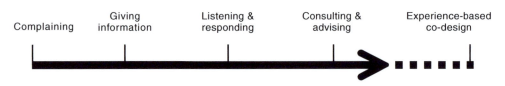

Figure 1.2   The continuum of patient influence. *Source*: Bate and Robert.[13]

prefix, suggesting more of a partnership and shared leadership, with NHS staff continuing to play a key role in leading service design but alongside patients and users. At the same time it does not mean trying to make patients and users into healthcare or design 'experts', but having them there *because* they are patients – 'lead users' rather than leaders – with that precious and very special kind of knowledge we call the first-hand experience of a service.

This type of approach means that designing 'systems', 'pathways' and 'processes' – concepts which have dominated health service design and redesign work for nearly a decade, and the field of total quality management (TQM) for nearly three decades – will need to move over and make some room for the experience concept. It is not a question of replacing them – as we shall see there will still be as great a need as ever for process mapping, care pathways and other well-established methods and tools – but of expanding and enriching the concept of service improvement, and with it our storehouse of methods and techniques.

There is a wealth of new material out there in the design sciences and, wider still, in the philosophy and ethnography of experience, that has the potential to take healthcare service improvement in some new and exciting directions, and that will help to shape the next generation of improvement methods and processes. These are the sources we shall be tapping into in this book.

Aims of the book

The overall aim of this book is to begin to open up and share some of that wealth with healthcare audiences and thus open up the prospect of big improvements in quality of care.

Taking as its reference the move towards the prioritisation of 'user experience' in both the culture and the design practices of service organisations (and similar, though less advanced, trends in this direction in healthcare and wider society), our book sets out to achieve four broad objectives:

1   to examine healthcare quality and service improvement challenges from the fresh angle of contemporary design and the service design professions, a process which will involve the exploration of new concepts, methods, and practices, most of which are currently outside the health field
2   to draw the attention of improvement researchers and practitioners in particular to the multidisciplinary field of interactive or 'user-centric design' and the whole concept of 'co-designing for user experience'
3   to take the concepts of user involvement and user experience and make them the focus of a different, and more intense, kind of attention in order to discover ways of *seeing deeper into experience*, of appreciating why it is important to be 'designing experiences' and not just systems or processes, and

4   to interest and equip readers with sufficient information, interest and understanding to go out and get involved in the 'doing' of EBD.

In doing this, we shall be drawing upon a range of methods, from literature
reviews to primary case studies and action research, trying as we go to get a judicious balance between research and practice, and to ensure that the necessary
translation occurs between them. We have always had the ambition of seeing
'more researching practitioners and more practising researchers' and hope that
this book goes some way to achieving this two-way flow in the field in question.

References

1   Berry LL, Wall EA, Carbone LP. Service clues and customer assessment of the service
    experience: lessons from marketing. *Academy of Management Perspectives*. 2006; **20**(2):
    43–57.
2   Farah S. Experience preferred. *CMO Magazine*. 2005; November. www.cmomagazine.
    com/read/110105/experience.html (accessed 11 September 2006).
3   Berry LL, Bendapudi, N. Clueing in customers. *Harvard Business Review*. 2003; February
    reprint R0302H.
4   Galbraith JR. *Designing the Customer-centric Organization. A Guide to Strategy, Structure and
    Process*. San Francisco: Jossey-Bass; 2005.
5   Pearse J. Review of patient satisfaction measures and experience surveys for public
    hospitals in Australia. www.pc.gov.au/gsp/reports/consultancy/patientsatisfaction/
    index.html (accessed 5 September 2006).
6   Department of Health. *The NHS in England: The Operating Framework for 2006/07*.
    London: TSO; 2006.
7   Schoen S, Osborn R, Trang P *et al*. Taking the pulse of health care systems: experiences
    of patients with health problems in six countries. *Health Affairs*, web exclusive. 3
    November 2005; W5–509-W5–525. www.cmwf.org/publications/publications_show.
    htm?doc_id=313012&#doc313 (accessed 3 November 2005).
8   Bate SP, Robert G, Bevan H. The next phase of health care improvement: what can we
    learn from social movements? *Quality and Safety in Health Care*. 2004; **13**(1): 62–6.
9   McGlynn EA, Asch SM, Adams J *et al*. The quality of health care delivered to adults in
    the United States. *New England Journal of Medicine*. 2003; **348**(26): 2635–45.
10 Institute of Medicine. *Crossing The Quality Chasm: A New Health System for the 21st
    Century*. Washington, DC: Institute of Medicine; 2001.
11 Australian Council for Safety and Quality in Health Care. *Patient Safety: Towards Sustainable
    Improvement. Fourth Report to the Australian Ministers' Conference*. Sydney: Commonwealth
    of Australia; 2003.
12 Department of Health. *The Way Forward. The NHS Institute for Learning, Skills and
    Innovation*. London: TSO; 2005.
13 Bate SP, Robert G. Experience-based design: from redesigning the system around the
    patient to co-designing services with the patient. *Quality and Safety in Health Care*. 2006;
    15(5): 307–10.
14 Berkun S. Programmers, designers and the Brooklyn Bridge. Essays on design, engi-
    neering and project management. 2004. www.scottberkun.com/essays/essay30.htm
    (accessed 7 December 2006).
15 Petit-Zeman S. *Doctor, What's Wrong? Making the NHS Human Again*. Abingdon: Routledge;
    2005.
16 Keaveney SM. Customer switching behaviour in service industries: an exploratory
    study. *Journal of Marketing*. 1995; **59**(2): 71–82.
17 Bate SP, Robert G. Choice. More could mean less (editorial). *British Medical Journal*.
    2005; **331**: 1488–9.

18 Berry LL, Parasuraman A, Zeithaml VA. Improving service quality in America: lessons learned. *Academy of Management Executive.* 1994; **8**(2): 32–44.

19 National Audit Office. *A Safer Place for Patients: Learning to Improve Patient Safety. Report by the Comptroller and Auditor General.* London: TSO; 2005.

20 Rettig M. Interface design when you don't know how. *Communication of the ACM.* 1992; **35**(1): 29–34.

21 Marcus A. *Graphic Design for Electronic Documents and User Interfaces.* New York: ACM Press/Addison-Wesley; 1991.

22 Scheiderman B. *Designing the User Interface.* Reading, MA: Addison-Wesley; 1987.

23 Gadney M. The secret of making things work. http://news.bbc.co.uk/1/hi/magazine/4393468.stm (accessed 11 September 2006).

24 Hudspith S. Utility, ceremony, and appeal: a framework for considering whole product function and user experience. *DRS News* (electronic version). 1997.

25 IDEO. S500 for 3M CDI. Blood parameter measurement system. www.ideo.com/portfolio/re.asp?x=50010 (accessed 4 August 2006).

26 Arnold K. Programmers are people, too. *Security.* 2005; **3**(5). www.acmqueue.com/modules.php?name=Content&pa=printer_friendly&pid=3 (accessed 30 August 2005).

27 Department of Health. *Creating a Patient-Led NHS. Delivering the NHS Improvement Plan.* London: TSO; 2005.

28 Department of Health. *Autumn Performance Report.* London: TSO; 2004.

29 Berkowitz B, Wolff T. *The Spirit of Coalition.* Washington, DC: American Public Health Association; 2000.

30 Green L, Mercer SL. Can public health researchers and agencies reconcile the push from funding bodies and the pull from communities? *American Journal of Public Health.* 2001; **91**: 1926–9.

31 Minkler M, Wallerstein N, editors. *Community-Based Participatory Research for Health.* New York, NY: Jossey-Bass; 2003.

32 Viswanathan M, Ammerman A, Gartlehner G *et al.* Community-based participatory research: a summary of the evidence on research methodology and community involvement. Poster presentation at the 6th International Conference on the Scientific Basis of Health Services; 2005 Sep 18–20; Montreal, Canada.

33 Cottam H, Leadbeater C. *RED Report 01. Health: Co-Creating Services.* London: The Design Council; 2004

34 Murray R, Burns, C, Vanstone C *et al. RED Report 01. Open Health.* London: The Design Council; 2005.

35 Pine BJ, Gilmore JH. *The Experience Economy.* Boston, MA: Harvard Business School Press; 1999.

36 Schmitt BH. *Customer Experience Management: A Revolutionary Approach to Connecting With Your Customers.* San Francisco, CA: Wiley; 2003.

37 Alben L. Quality of experience: defining the criteria for effective interaction design. *Interactions.* 1996; **3**(3): 11–15.

Part 1

Concepts

Our first part (Chapters 2–4) introduces the two major conceptual themes that run throughout this book: design and experience. Chapter 2 outlines the 'quiet revolution' that has been taking place in the design sciences by exploring the methods used by the design professions (like architects and software designers) and how such professions have come to see 'co-design' and 'experience' as crucial to their work. Chapter 3 specifies how a co-design approach markedly differs in at least five ways from the process redesign and re-engineering techniques normally found in healthcare quality and service improvement efforts (and their associated approaches to 'user involvement'). Chapter 4 then delves deeper into the nature and meaning of 'experience' and how others (especially anthropologists) have sought to make sense out of how people experience their lives. This chapter ends with a discussion of (a) resolving the difficulties of defining and explaining 'experience' (using phenomenology – 'the science of experience' – as its starting point) and (b) the remaining challenges facing those seeking to implement an EBD approach.

Chapter 2

A quiet revolution in design

Understanding experience is a critical issue for a variety of professions, especially design. (Jodi Forlizzi and Katja Battarbee)

The most important concept to grasp is that all experiences are important and that we can learn from them. (Nathan Shedroff)

No man's knowledge can go beyond his experience. (John Locke)

Placing the user of a service or a product at the very heart of the design process – what recently has been described as the 'quiet revolution in design'[1] – has become today's 'big idea' in professions such as architecture, computer, building, product, graphic and service design. On the whole this must be good news, for up until now the rhetoric of user involvement, including within healthcare itself, has been running some steps ahead of its practice. Even as we write in the summer of 2006 several national newspapers have been running the headline: 'Health forums "ailing"', describing how 'patients' forums are failing to achieve their aim of scrutinising health services and influencing policy and practice at a local level because they are being hamstrung by weak structures and are mired in bureaucracy and administration (*The Guardian*, 11 May 2006).

These concerns are not unfounded. As two recent official reports[2,3] found, the NHS is still not putting patients first, and despite improvements wide variations continue to exist between different services and organisations. The Healthcare Commission report,[2] the more recent of the two, states that the health service could still often seem to be designed around the needs of NHS staff rather than patients. The Commission chairman, Sir Ian Kennedy, said there was much for the health service to celebrate but added:

> *The government has set itself the aim of a 'patient-led NHS'. But our health services still have a long way to go before we can say that they are really putting patients first. Being an NHS patient is too often a frustrating experience.*[4]

In a similar vein, another report also bemoaned the lack of progress towards real patient involvement in service design, especially at the local, clinical microsystem level:

> *So far, developments have focused mainly on macro-level participation, and although the quality of face-to-face relationships is difficult to measure, progress towards empowerment, the sharing of power, increased patient choice and patient-centred care appears less well advanced . . . Further work is needed to establish what goes on in individual, face-to-face clinical encounters, and the extent to which stakeholders are taking forward an agenda of patient-centred care appears less well advanced.*[5]

While this report blamed the lack of progress on the persistence of medical paternalism, significantly we believe it still smacked of the traditional mindset that conceives of professional stakeholders taking up patient issues on behalf of the patients rather than letting the patients take them up for themselves as co-designers within a design process. In contrast to this conventional perspective, this book will look not only at ways of bringing about more patient-centred care, but of how patients may become more active partners in the definition and design of that care.

Our reservations apart, a recently published international survey has added weight to the observation above by stating that 'progress towards patient-centred care appears less well advanced' in the UK (all the more so because this latest critique is based on patients' perceptions themselves[6]). While the UK came out in the middle of this six-country study overall on six domains, even achieving a flattering first in patients' rankings on equity and safety perceptions, it only managed fourth out of six on patients' perceptions of 'patient-centredness', with Germany, New Zealand and Australia coming higher in the rankings (*see* Figure 2.1).

A larger study – but this time based solely on secondary data – across 25 European countries placed the United Kingdom in 15th place overall (behind Hungary, Malta and Slovenia among others) in terms of the user-friendliness of each country's healthcare system;[7] the survey was scored according to five 'sub-disciplines' (patients' rights and information; waiting times for treatment; outcomes; provision levels; and pharmaceuticals). On this occasion France came top, with the Netherlands and then Germany in second and third place.

To counter this somewhat depressing picture, some readers might feel compelled to point to the fact that, with the recent establishment of a new national system of patient and public involvement, which includes patient and public involvement forums, and patient advice and liaison services (PALS) in every NHS trust, independent complaints advocacy services (ICAS), a new Commission for Patient and Public Involvement in Health, and a new Director for Patient and Public Involvement within the Department of Health, things can only get better. Certainly this is the official view,[8] but even here there are no guarantees. For example, a recent in-depth academic study of PALS services in London[9] revealed that their role was more one of short-term problem-solving than longer-term

	AUS	CAN	GER	NZ	UK	US
Overall Ranking	4	5	1	2	3	6
Patient Safety	4	5	2	3	1	6
Effectiveness	4	2	3	6	5	1
Patient-Centeredness	3	5	1	2	4	6
Timeliness	4	6	1	2	5	3
Efficiency	4	5	1	2	3	6
Equity	2	4	5	3	1	6
Health Expenditures per Capita*	$2,903	$3,003	$2,996	$1,886	$2,231	$5,635

Note: 1=highest ranking, 6=lowest ranking.
* Health expenditures per capita figures are adjusted for differences in cost of living.
Health expenditures data are from 2003, except UK data (2002).

Figure 2.1 Patients' reports on care experiences. *Source*: Davis and Schoen.[6]

service improvement or development, and their links – and hence the patients' links – with the organisation's wider change and improvement processes tenuous, to say the least.

From 'redesigning the system around the patient' to 'co-designing services with the patient'

Designing – or rather redesigning – healthcare processes from the patient perspective was a key theme in the NHS Plan[10] – 'our aim is to redesign the system around the patient' (para 6.4) – and led to the rapid growth of practical redesign initiatives throughout the NHS. These various initiatives had in common the aim of thinking through the best process to achieve speedy and effective care from a patient perspective.[11] However, while patient/user involvement has been around healthcare for a long time now, what it gains in longevity, it seems (to us at least) to have lost in vitality and urgency. The ground, and the language itself, often appear tired and the word 'patient-centred' has become almost as overworked as the words 'new and improved' on soap packets. Progress since the 2000 Plan, as already noted, has been patchy and slow.

In our view, addressing what is both a problem and a challenge requires some fresh energy sources, and this is where establishing links with wider design professions may have a role to play. Healthcare may sound a far cry from the worlds of computing and architecture, which indeed it is (and this makes it exciting in itself), but the one thing that unites those most unlikely groups of professionals is simply their passion to make it 'better' for the user. Furthermore, they seek to achieve this by making that user integral to the design process itself, focusing on his or her *experience* of moving through the service and interacting with its various parts. Consider for example the eloquent words of one of today's leading designers and architects, Frank Gehry:

> *Without the client, you're one hand, you're the sound of one hand clapping. The client is the variable, and if the client engages with you, that's the opportunity.*[12]

And then ask: is it or should it be any different for the 'client' or user of a healthcare system? We find it difficult to find any reason why it should be.

Any opportunity for closing the gap between the preach and practice of patient-centred care must, in our view, be welcomed, especially when it suggests going beyond the token involvement of a user on some group or other, safely removed from the real scene of the action, to something approaching direct user engagement and participation – involvement and inclusion being very different both in concept and in practice. On the other hand, we have seen this all before and are rightly suspicious of anything that promises too much, or smacks of bandwagons and fast-buck commercialism (and it is true that many design firms today *are* already unashamedly marketing 'user-based design' as their USP (unique selling point)). In her classic book *Philosophy in a New Key*, Susanne Langer observes that certain ideas regularly burst upon the landscape with tremendous force, promising to resolve everything.[13] Not surprisingly everyone snaps them up as today's 'open sesame', and runs around excitedly telling others all about these ideas and enrolling them as guinea pigs or converts in their intellectual experiments. Fortunately, it does not take long to discover that the 'grand idée' is not so grand after all, does not explain or solve all, or even some, of the problems, or work in every situation, and therefore that it is time to move on to the next big idea!

It is anyone's guess as to how big this particular big idea – EBD – is or how long it will last, but what is certain is that it would be a pity if it were to come and go, simply passing healthcare by without due note or consideration. This is particularly true given the contemporary healthcare context in England as represented by the recent Department of Health publication, *Creating a Patient-Led NHS: Delivering the NHS Improvement Plan*.[14] This significant policy document sets out the ambition:

> to change the whole system so that there is more choice, more personalised care, real empowerment of people to improve their health – a fundamental change in our relationships with patients and the public . . . to move from a service that does things to and for its patients to one which is patient led, where the service works with patients to support them with their health needs.[14]

Clearly this is a place where the design professions might make a contribution, not least in challenging some of the assumptions underlying today's rhetoric of a 'patient-led NHS' itself and some of the methods and approaches that accompany it.

This brings us to the first broad aim of this book, which is simply to draw the attention of healthcare improvement policy makers and professionals to the burgeoning and, we think, exciting multidisciplinary field of interactive or 'user-centric design' and to the whole concept of 'co-designing for user experience'. In going there, we believe it will not only be a case of finding new, and sometimes very different, concepts, models, methods and processes for service development which a different kind of improvement professional has been working on – which there are in rich and creative abundance, and who will not disappoint – but also of tapping into the energy and passion that accompany any contemporary big idea when people begin to experiment with, and seek to stretch, exploit and extend it in different directions. The underlying idea is a very simple one but nevertheless has strong and profound resonances for healthcare. Just as many of today's designers have moved from designing inanimate objects like a glass to thinking about and designing the experience of drinking from that glass, so too, we shall argue, must healthcare improvement practitioners now begin to move from designing inanimate things like care processes to designing the experience of moving through that process. The beauty of this is that one is inevitably drawn back to the 'object' itself – the difference being, however, that it will now be the experience driving the design of the object rather than the other way round.

Tapping into the design professions

So where is this new and growing community of practice to be found? Unfortunately, this is not easy to answer. Its members appear under a plethora of different professional headings, and do not carry any common calling card or subscribe to any unified theory. Hence – just for starters – we are likely to encounter on this particular journey participatory design (PD), interactive or interaction design, empathetic design, human-centred design (and its sub-specialism 'human–computer interaction' (HCI)), usability engineering, high interactivity design, co-design, co-creation, co-operative interaction, co-operative design, participatory action research, people-centred design (PCD), user-based design, interactive design, user-centric/centred design (UCD), user experience design (UX or UXD), and experience (based) design (ED). Key in any of these words on a web search engine, and thousands of special interest groups, conferences, consultancies, journals and papers will soon be crowding your screen, all of them claiming to be into the same big idea and 'emerging paradigm' of designing *with* and *for* the user. Clearly the 'for the user' part already features strongly in the current 'patient-led' discourse found within NHS documents, so in a sense the fields already overlap and have much in common. The 'with the user' part is less advanced in the NHS, however, and while there has always been a concern to 'listen' to patients and users, and to give them third-party representation, this has generally stopped short of direct involvement in the co-design of services.

Despite the thousands of results from the web search above, it does not take long to find the four main watering holes where people of this particular persuasion tend to congregate. The only truly dedicated multidisciplinary EBD places are the Experience Designer Network (*see* http://experiencedesignernetwork.com), and 'Gel' (Good Experience Live, www.goodexperience.com) which consist of multidisciplinary groups of designers, journalists, planners and futurists that meet regularly, and have their own regular journal publications and e-newsletter exchanges. The other two occupy space within larger fields such as computing, which has its own professional association (ACT) and a special interest group on interactive design (and with a particular focus on human–computer interaction); and architecture which has the equivalent in the American Institute for Graphic Arts, and similar specialist groups on interactive and experience design. In the light of this, several commentators have suggested (rightly in our view) that it would be better to view experience design as a somewhat loose multidisciplinary community (communities?) of practice rather than a single tight profession. We view this as being broadly a positive thing because it implies a melting pot of professionals and professions and no single group or discipline hogging it all to itself. The fact that the term refers to experience rather than a particular professional or disciplinary group like graphic designers is encouraging in itself because it suggests a willingness to work in multiple design disciplines. A good example of this is a group which brings architecture, technology and architecture together; it has its own peer-written journal *Boxes and Arrows* which features many articles on experience-based and participatory design (*see* www.boxesandarrows.com). That being said, a community of practice for experience design still seems some way off, for, as Jacobson pointed out, despite everything, designers still tend to be extremely parochial, and not good at communicating outside their professional silos, even when they share the same commitment to things like experience design.[15] The fortunate thing here is that healthcare experience designers would be joining a community that is still very much in formation and therefore all the more open to newcomers.

Arguably there is another group that needs to be added in here, namely organisation researchers. This consists of people who, like us, have been drawn to the paradigm of design and the design sciences because of the potential it has for enriching our own field, especially in helping to heal the 'research into practice' divide which has had the effect of reducing the relevance and utility of much of their work, while at the same time advancing the theory and practice of organisational change and improvement. For readers who are interested, Boland and Collopy provide a recent literature review and overview of this burgeoning field of endeavour.[16] A number of the people currently using design approaches and methods within the NHS, including the present authors, arrived there via the organisation studies (OS) rather than the design route, notably through the pioneering work of OS design academics like George Romme and Joan van Aken (cited with others in Bate and Robert[17]). Boland and Collopy's DVD film of a unique conference that brought together designers such as Frank Gehry with organisation academics like Karl Weick for a learning exchange has been a source of inspiration to many.[18] Galbraith's guide to *Designing the Customer-Centric Organization*[19] is a further manifestation of the growing awareness that all organisations must increasingly strive to 'organise around the customer'. Pursuing the OS–design sciences link, a special issue of the *Journal of Applied Behavioral Science* on 'Bringing the design sciences to organisational development and change management' (editor SP Bate) has been commissioned for early 2007, and a similar issue of *Organisation Studies* for 2008. We mention these because they suggest a field of inquiry that is currently fizzing with new ideas, theories and practices.

Defining the field: designing the user experience

As might be expected there are the usual differences between the various schools and professions involved in both frame of reference and field of application, but these are more than outweighed by the similarities between them, not least their unswerving commitment to the direct involvement of users in designing their own experiences. It is therefore possible to put a general definition around the field, albeit by way of a collage of fragments culled from various sources (*see* Box A).

Box A: The participatory 'co' aspect of experience-based design

'Systems design for, with, and by the users.' (Briefs, Ciborra and Schneider, 1983)

   'Participatory Design (PD) makes users part of the design team and in this way can the design get immediately altered by first-hand experiences and we can more directly design artefacts that fill real needs and desires.' (Tollmar, 2004: p. 3)

   'The social inclusion and active participation of the people who use the services.' (numerous)

   'A set of diverse ways of thinking, planning and action through which people make their work technologies and social institutions more responsive to human needs.'

   'Participatory Design aims at including the future users in the design . . . in order to change the design . . . for the better.' (Dittrich, 2003)

   'Newer approaches that encourage creative thinking and doing design as participatory work between users and designers, making it more likely that the finished product or service will have the functionality required and work as the user envisions.' (Stanford University)

'Users play a central role in participatory design sessions, telling us about their work environments and the tasks they're trying to accomplish, including what works for them and what doesn't when they use their current tools.' (Tec-Ed, consultant to companies such as Sun Microsystems, Cisco Systems and Logitech)

'The goal is to provide a context for design experts where they can gain the practical understanding they need for successful design. Users possess the needed practical understanding but lack the insight designers have into new technical possibilities . . . Design takes on new meaning in participatory design as the interaction between practical understanding and creation.' (Stanford University)

Of course, as Shedroff rightly points out, such interactivity is nothing new.[20] People have been interacting with each other for as long as they have existed. What *is* new is that we consider it possible for computers, buildings, even services, to be interactive; that is, for people to truly *interact* with these things not just to *use* them. That being said, technologies, commodities and services are not inherently or automatically interactive: 'they must be made so through careful development that makes a place for the audience (users) to take part in the action'.[20] The role of participatory or interactive design is to construct opportunities and processes for just that thing to happen.[21]

One point about this role (and the source of some confusion, not to say self-delusion) needs to be understood from the outset; 'experience' can be supported by or influenced through design but never wholly controlled by it. Anyone who is a control freak or prefers top-down change should therefore probably stay away from EBD. Jane Fulton Suri makes the point nicely, at the same time giving strong clues as to why EBD can never be entirely deterministic or prescriptive but at best a partnership in which designers and users come together to *co-design* a product or service:

> *Experience itself is personal and, though designers can influence it, it cannot be designed. Indeed many aspects of experience – those affected by people's internal states, moods and idiosyncratic associations or by context – are independent of designers' control. But experience is also influenced by factors that designers do control: the formal sensory qualities, sound, feedback, rhythm, sequence, layering and logic – all the expressive qualities inherent in the products, environments, media and services we design.*[22]

Forlizzi says very much the same thing when she points out that 'we can't really design an experience, only the mechanisms for creating it, and the interactive and expressive behaviours that modulate experience'.[23]

This brings us to another aim of this book, which is all to do with that somewhat overworked phrase 'making the familiar strange': we want to take this concept of 'the patient experience', or wider 'the user experience', and make it the focus of a different, and more intense, kind of attention. We want to put it centre-stage, train the spotlight on it, illuminate it, and examine it more closely. The academic term for this is 'bracketing'; blowing a concept's cover of 'normalness', which in this book actually began the minute we put speech marks around the word 'experience', thereby pulling it out of the stream of unremarked, everyday use. The aim in doing this is, quite simply, to discover ways of *seeing deeper into experience*, of appreciating why it is so much more important to be 'designing experiences' than just systems or processes, and to be engaging with it head on, rather than treating it as the backdrop to design.

Targeting 'experience'

We shall suggest that designing services, environments, interactions and processes for the human experience – literally 'targeting experience' – poses a formidable, but highly worthwhile, challenge for healthcare improvement professionals. This is not just about being more 'patient-centred' or promoting greater 'patient involvement'. It goes much further than this in completely reorienting the improvement process around patients' and users' 'experience goals', placing them at the heart of the design process, and on as – or more – important a footing as process and clinical goals. The nature of the challenge is to understand their experience of care at a deep level, always bearing in mind that it includes all aspects of experiencing a product or service – physical, sensual, cognitive, kinetic, aesthetic and above all emotional (the notion of the patient journey as an emotional as well as clinical experience) – and to use this understanding to design a healthcare experience that will be more 'successful' and 'satisfying' than it has ever been before.

'Experience' is personal, whereas systems are abstract and impersonal, and in a way, that is the only reality that matters in design, indeed in life itself. We can illustrate this point quite simply by reflecting on what are widely recognised as 'good' experiences (using Google or Amazon, for example) or that all-too-familiar example of a 'bad experience' of design (*see* Figure 2.2), which might equally be expressed as an experience of 'bad design'.

Many readers will identify with that feeling of panic when, just minutes before your PowerPoint presentation is about to begin, you find that you can't get your laptop to synchronise with the projector! At this point, there is nothing more important in the world than getting beyond the blue 'no signal' warning message, or worse, the blank screen, and yet instead of using those precious last few moments to get your head around what you are about to say, you find yourself struggling with an array of 'stupid' wires, connections and buttons that, no matter where you connect them or what order you press them, stubbornly refuse to give you what you want. As Martin, whose example this is,[24] says, what is the point of a high-tech piece of equipment if you can't turn it on? The point – imperative – for designers, including health service designers, is to focus on designing experiences that at the very least do not induce fear, anxiety, confusion, uncertainty or panic in the user (and at best are smooth, natural and trouble-free, and look and feel good), since to all intents and purposes there is no reality beyond that experience, and nothing more important at the time than the way it – that interaction – feels. What is interesting in this case, though not at all untypical, is that the designers designed a piece of technology that on our three elements of good design would probably score 10 out of 10 for functionality (in terms of a huge range of things it can do) and reliability (bulbs these days rarely blow) but in the event came in at zero on the interactivity and usability aspects covered by the third element, the aesthetics of experience. The same can equally

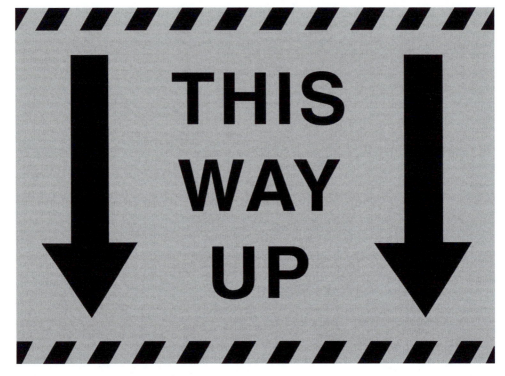

Figure 2.2   A 'bad experience' of design.

apply to a service, like healthcare. The most perfectly designed treatment pathway in the world can still be a disaster from an experience point of view.

All of us will have our own personal examples of such 'experience sinks' and design stupidities – computers and telephone systems that have frustrating features and functions, mobile phones that perversely make a noise when you want to switch them off and render them silent, companies that offer a call desk facility you can never access (condemning you to an endless loop of Vivaldi's *Four Seasons, Spring*), cameras, supermarkets, airports and hospitals that seem to have been deliberately designed to give you, the user, a hard time. By citing these many examples of bad design we are also seeking to avoid the familiar trap of lionising or adulating designers, acknowledging that they can indeed be just as stupid as the rest of us. For some wonderful everyday examples of bad design, *see* Michael Darnell on www.baddesigns.com/, one of whose latest humorous offerings is the Keanall Portable Charcoal Grill Model KD300 whose manufacturers chose to paint the barbeque with flammable paint! For us, one of the funniest examples we have encountered, and a useful counterbalance to the seriousness that follows, is one of the great breakthroughs in design, the square lavatory seat! This appeared on the www.thisisbroken.com website, which is also dedicated to such design stupidities. The victim described it as follows: 'Here is a picture [Figure 2.3] of the toilet in my London hotel. The toilet is square. My butt, like most, is round. In the presence of so many alternative designs that provide a better experience, this is a backwards innovation into brokenness.' On the other hand, it does remind us that good design always starts at the bottom!

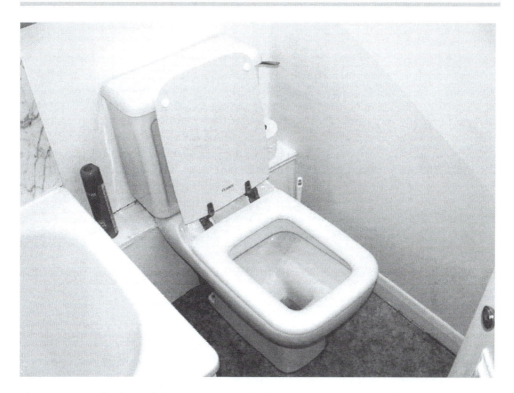

Figure 2.3   A backwards innovation into brokenness. *Source*: www.thisisbroken.com.

Bad design does not discriminate between products and services, and can be found anywhere and everywhere one cares to look, including a heathcare service. And there is really no excuse for this, in that the elements that contribute to superior experiences are knowable and reproducible, and, in this regard, designable.[25,26]

Having said that, we need to be constantly on our guard against what Davis has dubbed the 'right wing' of experience design:[27] the zealots who are attracted to a new idea like moths to light, whose agenda is control and manipulation and altered states of consciousness in their subjects. This is the 'engineered experience', as opposed to the designed experience, epitomised in the classic 1970s Yul Brynner film *Westworld* where sex, adventure, even death itself, could be simulated, albeit ultimately with disastrous consequences. Davis claims we have seen a dramatic rise in similar adrenalin-charged 'engineered experiences' in the past 15 years, such as bungee jumping, 'don't try this at home' gameshows, and exotic holiday experiences like guzzling ayahuasca with Peruvian shamans, caving in Belize or living with real monks in Bhutan. A line has been crossed from 'designed' into the plastic 'manufactured' experience, although it is never easy to actually pinpoint where that line is, and when one needs to take a step back. That being said, as has been observed elsewhere, perhaps people like Davis are overestimating the amount of control that designers may have over someone else's experience, and are misguided in implying that organisation designers have the same control over life and death as the bungee managers have! At the same time it all underlines the importance of having the 'co' or participatory element within

EBD, which helps to ameliorate the danger of an experience being designed for and imposed on the user.

In all of the cases cited above, good and bad, the lesson for designers is that they need to be designing not only a product or a service, but a total cognitive–emotional experience, which requires cultivated insight into, and appreciation of, people's fundamental human needs, hopes, fears and aspirations.[28] The 'North Star' is obviously the 'good experience', and we all know what that is when we encounter it. Stated simply, the good experience is, and should be, the ambition of design.

Enter the field of 'experience' (ED) or *experience*-based' (EBD) design, which two of its leading advocates in architecture have described as follows:

> *Designing for user experience – a process that involves developing 'service dialogues' with the user, the goal being 'to make experience accessible to the designers, to allow them to conceive of designing experiences rather than designing services'.*[23]

> *Experience is designated as 'how well people understand it, how they feel about it while they are using it, how well it serves its purpose, and how well it fits into the context in which they are using it'.*[29]

As we push beyond these introductory definitions, we will need to be absolutely clear as to what experience means in this context, as it can so easily become confused with neighbouring but very different concepts like 'perception' or 'attitude', or getting patients' 'views' about the service they receive (for example, surveys get at attitudes, but we would argue strongly that they do not often 'get at' experiences). 'Experience' is this and more. It is actually not so much an attitude as a particular, and very special, kind of *knowledge*, acquired from close personal observation or direct contact with something like a product, process, system or service – *personal knowledge*. The task for EBD is to gain access to that unique and precious form of knowledge and utilise it in the service of a better design, and a better experience for the user. That knowledge is expressed in what one thinks, feels and says about the experience of a service, process or product one has encountered. To explain *why* someone thinks or feels that way, for example why something like a particular brand of car or watch, or equally one's experience of attending a diabetes clinic, looks and feels 'good' (or not), requires an understanding of the interaction and relationship between the user and the service or product (for example, the human–computer or human–X-ray interactions we have already mentioned). If that relationship can be disentangled and understood, then it can begin to be shaped to look, feel and be better, hence the notion of 'designing for improvement'.

Understanding and designing material and physical goods like cars or computers around 'experiences' has been a major interest of designers and design writers for some time,[30,31] but less so in the case of 'services' such as healthcare. However, the factors determining emotional and cognitive reactions, and levels of satisfaction, are very similar, as are the elements that make up a good (user-friendly) or bad design. Consider, for example, the 'user-experience honeycomb' in Figure 2.4, created by experience designer Peter Morville, as a starter to what follows. This was initially produced for designing user-friendly computer software, but arguably, as with many of these models encountered in experience design, it might equally apply to the design of a hospital or healthcare services and interactions.

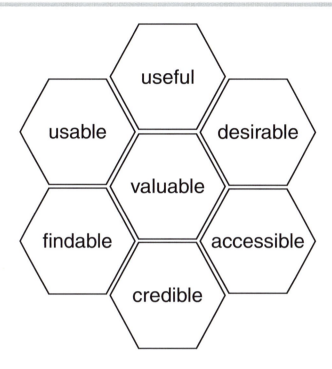

Where:

Useful   =   has practical value and serves a useful and needed purpose

Usable   =   ease and convenience of use (for example, access)

Desirable   =   emotionally and aesthetically attractive, appealing or satisfying

Findable   =   a service that is findable and navigable

Accessible =   to all kinds of people, young and old, able and disabled, with or without sensory, mobility or cognitive impairments (for example, magnifiers and braille keyboards on computers, and verbal announcements in lifts and railway systems for the blind)

Credible   =   a service and provider that is and can be trusted (clinically and managerially), and in whom we can believe

Valuable   =   must deliver value to all, most of all patients

Figure 2.4   User-experience honeycomb. *Source*: www.semanticstudios.com/publications/semantics/000029.php (accessed 18 September 2006). Reproduced with permission of Peter Morville, Semantic Studios LLC.

In many instances, products or services simply do not measure up on some, or indeed any, of these elements – for example, the service is not easy to find, or particularly desirable or successful once found. Findability was at the forefront of the Google project, and it does tempt one to ask which is it easiest to find one's way around, the boundless universe of knowledge or one's local hospital? The implication is that a service needs to be scrutinised every step of the way to ensure that 'experience' criteria like these are being met, and the overall 'usability' of the service is being constantly monitored – and here this begs the question why, given its importance and close connection to safety and reliability issues, 'usability' is not a major criterion in healthcare clinical governance considerations. Usability has been defined as the effectiveness, efficiency, and satisfaction users have with a service or product. 'High usability' has been defined in many different ways but generally means a system is: easy to learn and remember, efficient, easy and fun to use, and quick to recover from errors.[32] Obviously, the aspiration is a 'high usability' service that scores consistently highly on all these criteria for the full duration of the experience.

'Usability' is one area where healthcare services are still falling down badly. For example, Nielsen, a designer, recently reviewed[33] a study published in the *Journal of the American Medical Association*.[34] This study reported on 22 ways that automated hospital systems can result in the wrong medication being dispensed to patients. Most of these flaws are classic usability problems that have been understood for decades. All of these flaws existed, and remained uncorrected, says Nielsen, because of the failure of healthcare designers to be aware or reap the benefit of the last 25 years' experience with usability/interactivity research. More worrying, by relying on a questionnaire survey (of staff on this occasion) rather than observing actual experience, this particular study – he suggests – may have significantly underestimated the true error rate. His comments and the study itself are disturbing, and one is left to speculate on the proportion of design efforts in healthcare, even those that purport to 'listen' to users, that are failing to uncover potentially fatal processes.

In the particular model shown in Figure 2.4, usability is just one of the factors in user-experience, but more often the term is used to describe how useful, usable and user-friendly a product or service is overall, embracing factors such as:

- utility (how useful is it?)
- learnability (how easy is it to learn to navigate my way through?)
- efficiency (how efficiently does it deal with my needs?)
- retainability (how long does it stay in the memory and how easy is it to recall?)
- errors (how safe and error-free?)
- satisfaction (how pleasing an experience?).

Clearly there are many different usability models to draw on, and both differences and similarities between them to which we need to return later with the aim of synthesising them into a model or models best suited to the particular context of health services.

Summary

This chapter has introduced the concept of EBD, describing where work is going on, and why we think this is important and relevant to healthcare, particularly with regard to the next generation of NHS improvement methods. We have begun to unpack what we mean by 'experience' and why it is important to put this at the centre of any design activity. In this sense the broad theme of this whole section is about the importance of being *mindful* of experience, and to build that mindfulness into everything we do as improvement specialists. If this sounds too abstract or esoteric, listen to what the CEO of Procter & Gamble recently said about the need to put design 'into the DNA' of his own company:

We have to create a great experience every time you touch the brand, and the design is a really big part of creating the experience and the emotion. We try to make [a customer's experience] better, but better in her *terms. If you stay focused on experiences, I think you will have a lower risk of designing something that may measure well in a lab but may not do well with the consumer. I want P&G to become the number-one consumer-design company in the world, so we need to be able to make it part of our strategy. We need to make it part of our innovation process.*[35]

It is easy to dismiss this as perhaps suitable for housecare products but not necessarily patients, but we shall argue to the contrary that being mindful of experience and also putting it into the DNA of the healthcare organisation is as, if not more, important, not least because there is a good deal more at stake here than the feel of the bubbles in the washing-up sink (although maybe the aim of creating a great experience every time the patient touches the service is not that silly).

In the next chapter we want to take a broad sweep over the subject of EBD, recognising that it is a number of different things: a paradigm, a discipline and field of enquiry, a community of practice, an approach, as well as a set of tools and methods. The aim will be to begin to equip readers with sufficient information on all of these to enable them to go out and get involved in the 'doing' of EBD.

Before digging in at the detailed level, however, we want to return to our opening formula of 'good design' (*see* Figure 1.1 on page 5) in order to get one last high-level overview of our subject, and the three basic things that healthcare service design should be aiming for:

Performance (P) + Engineering (E) + Aesthetics (A)

This will be our constant guide in what follows, the central contention already having been stated that good, indeed great, design possesses all three elements in different manifestations and combinations. Consider for example the three winners of the recent BBC2 *Culture Show*'s 'Great Britain design quest': Concorde, the London underground map, and the Spitfire. Not only were these ruthlessly functional, reliable and well engineered (in the middle case conceived and drawn) (P and E), each was also very 'beautiful' in terms of aesthetic and interactivity, and exemplary in terms of the user experience or usability (A). Whatever iconic products or buildings one cares to think of – the London Routemaster bus (a runner-up), a Lambretta scooter, a Coke bottle – the three basic ingredients remain broadly the same. The – on first sight unlikely – link with healthcare, we would argue, is that this broad formula applies to services, too. The quality of a cancer service, for example, will be a function of **P**, the core activity of how efficiently and effectively it does the job of treating the patient (waiting time, treatment plan, and treatment itself); of **E**, how safely it is discharged (no errors, no harm, safe, reliable; recent catastrophic radiotherapy overdoses are a salutary reminder of the importance of this element); and of **A**, how the whole interface/interaction between patient and service is fashioned and managed (how it feels, how it is all 'experienced'). Viewed from this 'good design' perspective, healthcare service design needs to attend simultaneously to all three, although unfortunately at present this is often far from the case. Frequent scenarios that will be familiar to readers are that E is missed out of design completely (being consigned to the governance rather than improvement silo of the organisation), or that P (scheduling, waits, pathways, performance, etc.) and E (clinical governance, audits, safety, etc.) are dealt with separately with little or no co-ordination between them.

Our final word on why we think this formula is so important to healthcare service design is that we feel it addresses not one but all three major challenges that face any service design effort: namely implementation (making it happen on the ground/seeing the design translated into practice), spread (diffusion of the new design), and sustainability (making it last; holding the gains). For example, we know from the above examples that a good or great design spreads like wild-fire and will also tend to last, or to put it another way, there is a simple theory here that says if you want an improvement in healthcare to spread and embed, then make sure all three ingredients of the P + E + A formula are present. The additional attraction so far as EBD and participatory design in particular are concerned is that they seem to be more effective than other design methods in achieving implementation, spread and sustainability. On the sustainability question, for example, Canny has recently concluded from his review of some of the great design achievements in the last 50 years – such as the personal computer, office information systems, the internet and mobile phone – that 'When you execute the human-centred design process well you get a design that endures for decades'.[36] This is the same argument that we shall be developing in relation to health service design: strive to design a service that scores high on P, E and A, and successful spread and sustainability will be all the more likely.

References

1 Carton S. A quiet revolution in design. 13 June 2001. www.clickz.com/experts/ad/lead_edge/article.php/842921 (accessed 4 August 2006).
2 Healthcare Commission. *State of Healthcare*. London: Healthcare Commission; 2005.
3 Commission for Health Improvement. *Unpacking the Patients' Experience: Variations in the NHS Patient Experience in England*. London: CHI; 2004.
4 NHS 'not putting patients first'. BBC News website. http://news.bbc.co.uk/1/hi/health/4692801.stm (accessed 2nd August 2006).
5 Gillespie R, Florin D, Gillam S. *Changing Relationships. Findings from the Patient-Involvement Project*. London: The King's Fund; 2002.
6 Davis K, Schoen C, Schoenbaum SC *et al*. *Mirror, Mirror on the Wall: An Update on the Quality of American Health Care Through the Patient's Lens*. New York: The Commonwealth Fund; 2004.
7 Health Consumer Powerhouse. *European Health Consumer Index*. Stockholm: Health Consumer Powerhouse; 2006.
8 Department of Health. *Patient and Public Involvement in Health: The Evidence for Policy Implementation*. London: TSO; May 2004.
9 Buchanan D, Abbott S, Bentley J *et al*. Let's be PALS: user-driven organisational change in healthcare. *British Journal of Management*. 2005; **16**(4): 315–28.
10 Department of Health. *The NHS Plan*. London: TSO; 2000.
11 Locock L. *Maps and Journeys: Redesign in the NHS*. Birmingham; Health Services Management Centre, University of Birmingham; 2001.
12 Gehry F. *Gehry Talks: Architecture and Process*. London: Thames & Hudson; 2003.
13 Langer S. *Philosophy in a New Key: A Study in the Symbolism of Reason, Rite, and Art*. 3rd ed. Boston, MA: Harvard University Press; 1957.
14 Department of Health. *Creating a Patient-Led NHS. Delivering the NHS Improvement Plan*. London: TSO; 2005.
15 Jacobson R. Experience design. 18 August 2000. www.alistapart.com/articles/experience (accessed 4 August 2006).

16 Boland RJ, Collopy F, editors. *Managing as Designing*. Stanford, CA: Stanford Business Books; 2004.

17 Bate SP, Robert G. Towards more user-centric organisational development: lessons from a case study of experience-based design. *Journal of Applied Behavioral Science*. 2007; **43**(1): 41–66.

18 Boland RJ, Collopy F. *Managing as Designing. Bringing the Art of Design to the Practice of Management*. (DVD film.) Information Design Studio, Weatherhead School of Management, Case Western Reserve University; 2004.

19 Galbraith JR. *Designing the Customer-Centric Organization. A Guide to Strategy, Structure and Process*. San Francisco: Jossey-Bass; 2005.

20 Shedroff N. Experience design: interactivity. www.webreference.com/authoring/design/expdesign/6.html (accessed 7 December 2006).

21 Schuler D, Namioka A. *Participatory Design. Principles and Practices*. Hillsdale: Erlbaum; 1993.

22 Fulton Suri J. The experience evolution: developments in design practice. *The Design Journal*. 2003; **6**(2): 39–48.

23 Forlizzi J. *Designing for Experience: An Approach to Human-Centered Design*. Master of Design in Interaction Design Thesis, Carnegie Mellon University; 1997.

24 Martin A. In a cold dark stall. *Innovation*. 2003; Summer: 32–5.

25 Shedroff N. *Experience Design*. Berkeley; CA: New Rides Publishing; 2001.

26 Shedroff N. Experience design. Designing the total experience. 21 June 2001. www.webreference.com/authoring/design/expdesign/8.html (accessed 30 January 2005).

27 Davis E. Experience design and the design of experience. 2000. www.techgnosis.com/experience.html (accessed 2 August 2006).

28 Ardill R. About experience design. 2005. www.design-council.org.uk/webdav/harmonise?Page/@id=42&Session/@id=D_nR999Pvd1iIP16nTDvBp&Document/@id=523 2 (accessed 4 August 2006).

29 Alben L. Quality of experience: defining the criteria for effective interaction design. *Interactions*. 1996; **3**(3): 11–15.

30 Norman DA. *The Design of Everyday Things*. London: Basic Books; 2002.

31 Norman DA. *Emotional Design: Why We Love (or Hate) Everyday Things*. London: Basic Books; 2004.

32 *See*: www.remedy.com/customers/dev_community/UserExperience/accessibility.htm (accessed 2 August 2006).

33 Nielsen J. Medical usability: how to kill patients through bad design. 2005. www.useit.com/alertbox/20050411.html (accessed 4 August 2005).

34 Koppel R, Metlay JP, Cohen A *et al*. Role of computerized physician order entry systems in facilitating medication errors. *Journal of the American Medical Association*. 2005; **293**(10): 1197–203.

35 What P&G knows about the power of design. Interview with CEO, AG Lafley. June 2005. www.fastcompany.com/magazine/95/design-qa.html (accessed 2 August 2006).

36 Canny J. The future of human–computer interaction. *Human Computer Interaction*. 2006; **4**(6): 1–4.

Chapter 3

So what's different?

Experience design is an emerging paradigm, a call for inclusion. (Bob Jacobson)

Some readers will be thinking, what's new or different in any of what has been said so far from, say, a focus group, patient forum, attitude survey or discovery interview? Surely, it is just another way of talking about 'getting closer in touch' with the patient, and what could possibly be new about that? To some extent they are right to think this way. There is no such thing as a completely new field. As it is in management trends[1,2] so it is in design – and every other sphere of human activity – that fads and fashions come and go; often there is a lot of re-packaging and re-labelling going on, but the core contents are indeed similar or the same. For instance, reviewers of earlier drafts of this work have rightly drawn attention to certain areas of healthcare where patients and families have partici-pated for years in service design, and where considerable depth of learning already exists. For example, we are grateful to James B Conway (Dana-Farber Cancer Institute, Boston) for directing our attention to a website on paediatric services which lists many bibliographic sources on participatory design.[3] The only thing we would offer in our defence is that while the participatory element is not entirely new, the experience focus is more so. Most of the works cited in this bib-liography do not make any explicit reference to experience; and involvement does not necessarily mean a focus on experience, tending to be more about deci-sion-making than experience-making. In any case, it is never a good idea to try and convince people in advance of the arguments and the data – any change of mind comes from seeing and then judging what is on offer. However, such reser-vations apart, it is worth trying to flag up in advance what we see as the five dif-ferences between where things are now and where they could be if concepts of user participation and EBD were incorporated into existing and future healthcare improvement efforts.[4]

First, we would acknowledge that there are currently many ways in which car-ers and patients can and do get their voices heard, from the complaints end of the spectrum through to direct or indirect involvement on user groups, patient forums, focus groups, and surveys of various kinds. But let us be clear: while admirable in itself, being 'responsive to patients' needs and listening to their views'[5,6] alone are not co-design processes, at least not as we shall be describing them. Nor is it just about 'being on the spot and resolving issues before they esca-late into problems', 'being better informed', or 'having more of a say'.[5,6] EBD is all this and more, since users are not only active partners in their care but also the designers of their care. Therefore, it is not a case of staff 'responding' to user needs; the users are already there in person to express those needs for themselves as part and parcel of the design process. EBD is about direct and active user participation in the design process itself – the notion of users as designers – be that for a specific part or for the whole of the treatment process. *EBD, therefore, is truly a joint venture, one that involves users and professionals acting as the co-designers of a service.* In its com-plete sense, users may be involved in every step of the design process from diag-nosis and needs analysis, through envisioning and model building, to prototyping and testing, implementing and evaluating. And in this process they do not just say things, they do things as well; and they do them in person, not through some third party.

At the same time, EBD is not about turning patients into professional designers. That is still best left to trained designers themselves. The role of users (and the value and justification for their being there) is to bring *the knowledge of their experience* to the table so that the designers can work with them to translate and build that knowledge into new and future designs. It is in the coming together of two knowledge systems – what cognitive scientists call 'folk' (everyday, experience-based) knowledge and 'expert' knowledge (specialist, discipline-based) – that the innovation process really begins to ignite and take off. This is also why EBD is different from various kinds of 'Expert Patient' initiative, since there is no presumption about turning the patient into a clinical, or for that matter any other kind of, expert. For example, the 'Expert Patient Programme' in England is a self-management course for patients with long-term conditions and is concerned with offering a toolkit of fundamental techniques that patients can undertake to improve their quality of life. EBD, in contrast, assumes that the only expertise users bring is themselves and their experiences. The 'folk–expert' distinction made here might also go some way towards allaying anxieties some designers have expressed from time to time that we may become so user-centric that we lose the edge of innovation and become overly driven by users rather than be guided by their needs.[7] Essentially, what we are talking about here is a partnership between expert and user, not a user takeover!

So, in terms of framing, imagine a 'participation continuum' (or flick back to Figure 1.2 on page 10) with 'complaints' and 'research and audit' of patient views towards the one end (low involvement) and direct participation in 'designing services' at the other (high involvement), with peer-to-peer sharing of experiences (for example, *see* the impressive website www.dipex.org, which anyone can access in order to read or watch films of patients' accounts of their illness and treatment), and representative 'participation in user groups and patient focus groups' more towards the middle. Writers on the NHS experience seem to agree that patient participation has become stuck at the low end and suggest that it is time to 'progress beyond gathering data on patient views and presenting it to relevant committees' and moving towards much closer contact between users and design professionals.[8] Clearly, EBD (high involvement/inclusion end) fits nicely with this growing demand for more extensive and more direct forms of user participation. Certainly, as things stand, we are still some way off the situation where (a) experience is the central concern and organising principle of healthcare improvement, and (b) patients and users sit down with management and clinical professionals on equal terms and have a direct input into the design of the services they receive. Ten years ago this would have been just the same in the case of product or service design, but would be inconceivable today for companies like Apple or Starbucks.

The second difference between current 'patient involvement' strategies and EBD is that the focus of the latter is not so much on user 'views', 'attitudes', 'needs' or 'perceptions' (although all come into it) as user *experiences* – creating not just a service but a whole experience that appeals on a cognitive and emotional level. Research is therefore focused on appreciating and understanding how people experience the service they receive (which is what then shapes attitudes and perceptions). In this sense, *the discovery process is more about sense-making and meaning construction than attitudes or perceptions.*

Third, getting at experiences is a specialised activity that needs to be learned and practised. At the very least it requires a basic *knowledge of and training in ethnographic methods and the related methods of contextual inquiry* (*see* Chapters 5 and 8). This is why today we find many experience designers with an anthropological or ethnographic background.[9–12] Without these methods, what often poses as experience research is actually little more than a conversation that anyone might have had, and words and stories without analytical frameworks do not speak for themselves. It also requires proximity to the immediacies of the lives to be studied that may not be possible or may be denied because of one's present status or position in the organisation. Seniority does not give that access, indeed may often militate against it.

Fourth, in interpreting experiences, the main challenge is to understand *how the interface between user and service is shaped*. Most traditional service improvement methods do not concern themselves with that relationship, believing that a process can mostly be designed as a 'black box' whose contents do not need to be known.

Finally – and obviously – one is *designing experiences*, not processes or systems or just the built environment (although all come into it, as a means to a better experience but not an end in itself). Traditionally, improving patient experience by 'design' in the NHS has meant asking users about what aspects of the physical environment they would like to see improved. For example, a report of how Accident & Emergency (A&E) environments for patients and staff have been improved was entitled '*Better patient experience by design*'.[13] Traditional process-mapping techniques and pathways development may be involved in EBD, but the main focus is upon what might be called the 'subjective pathway' (emotional or experience map) rather than the objective pathway. This objective pathway is often taken literally to mean the various steps, stages and activities that a patient goes through; the subjective pathway is concerned with how it was experienced – the events, people, and issues along that pathway which shaped the experience. (Later we discuss the concept of 'touch points' in the journey, that is to say key moments and places where experiences were formed.) To design an experience is to place much greater focus on the user than the steps in the process. The two are very different. One can have the perfect process (fast, efficient, no bottlenecks) or pathway (evidence-based), but an incredibly poor experience, or even a poor-quality process and pathway, and a reasonable or good experience. One wonders what is the point of a great process and a terrible experience, which is why we believe the balance needs to be restored to take greater account of the latter. This will only happen when we recognise that process redesign and process re-engineering were originally developed in product and assembly line organisations which did not have to think of the experiences its cars and fridges were having as they passed from one stage to another. Of course, everyone knows that a patient is a sentient being not a fridge, in which case our question is why has it taken so long to build 'experience' into the design equation, and why persist for so long with techniques that are concerned solely with speed and efficiency, but not experience?

References

1 Abrahamson E. Managerial fads and fashions: the diffusion and rejection of innovation. *California Management Review.* 1991; **16**: 586–612.

2 Abrahamson E, Fairchild G. Management fashion: life-cycles, triggers and collective learning processes. *Administrative Sciences Quarterly.* 1999; **44**: 708–40.

3 Bibliography and other resource materials for advancing patient- and family-centred care. Bethseda, MD: Institute for Family-Centred Care. www.familycenteredcare.org/advance/IFCC_Bibliography.pdf (accessed 4 August 2006).

4 Bate SP, Robert G. Experience-based design: from redesigning the system around the patient to co-designing services with the patient. *Quality and Safety in Health Care.* 2006; **15**(5): 307–10.

5 Department of Health. *The NHS Plan.* London: TSO; 2000.

6 Department of Health. *Shifting the Balance of Power Within the NHS.* London: TSO; 2001.

7 Malone E. AIGA Experience Design Summit #5. 16 July 2002. www.boxesandarrows.com/archives/aiga_experience_design_summit_5.php (accessed 2 August 2006).

8 Fisher B. *Patients as Teachers – 'What Works For You?' A New Way of Involving Users in Improving Services.* Unpublished paper on two 'patients as teachers' initiatives in Lambeth, Southwark and Lewisham Health Authority. 2005.

9 Hughes J, O'Brien J, Rodden T *et al.* Designing with ethnography: a presentation framework for design. *Proceedings of DIS '97 Designing Interactive Systems: Processes, Practices, Methods and Techniques.* Amsterdam: ACM Press; 1997.

10 Kantner L, Hinderer Sova D, Rosenbaum S. Alternative methods for field usability research. *Proceedings of SIGDOC.* San Francisco, CA: ACM Press; 2003.

11 Anschuetz L, Rosenbaum, S. Ethnographic interviews guide design of web site for vehicle buyers. *Proceedings of CHI.* New York: ACM Press; 2003.

12 Brooke T, Burrell J. From ethnography to design in a vineyard. *Proceedings of the Conference on Designing User Experiences.* New York: ACM Press; 2003.

13 Better patient experience by design. Modernising A & E Environments. NHS Estates. 6 April 2004. www.dh.gov.uk/PublicationsAndStatistics/PressReleases/PressReleasesNotices/fs/en?CONTENT_ID=4078971&chk=er8j2J (accessed 2 August 2006).

Chapter 4

The intellectual roots of experience design

Coming into the country, virtually any country . . . is an experience palpable enough to be felt on the skin, and penetrant enough to be felt beneath it. The difficulty lies in articulating that experience, making it available to common view. (Clifford Geertz)

The anthropological quest to represent the lives and experiences of others

'Experience-based' research and practice have their origins in both the design sciences and the social sciences, and anthropology in particular, which provides the root academic discipline for both domains. For instance, most experience-design firms like IDEO and FIORI Design in the US, and Flow-Interactive in the UK, have substantial numbers of anthropologists on their staff. Anthropology's defining quest – and the grounds upon which it originally set itself up as the opposition to 'objective' science – is to represent the lives and experiences of others,[1] to convey what it 'feels like' or 'looks like' *to you* (hence that old anthropologist's joke of 'I know how it was for you, but how was it for me?'). 'What is it like to work here or to be a patient here?' and similar types of open-ended questions are used to piece together how participants *made sense of it for themselves;*[2] their 'meanings in use',[3] this also being the aim of qualitative research in general (as Gephart[3] notes, 'Qualitative research addresses questions about how social experience is created and given meaning'). The anthropological commitment to seeing it from the actor's perspective is central to the doing of EBD, in fact to change practice of any kind, a point made by management writer Edgar Schein when recently looking back on his professional life:

In reflecting on [my own] practice . . . I have often found myself saying to practitioners in workshops that . . . they need to learn to think like an anthropologist, accepting culture for what it is, suspending judgement until they see it from the 'native point of view' . . .[4]

Hence the commitment is to going out and learning about the actors' world, *their* reality, what *they* make of it all; the view from the seat in the waiting room or under the MRI (magnetic resonance imaging) scanner (including the child's or the claustrophobic's), insider-out as opposed to outsider-in. The whole point of the anthropological or ethnographic quest, as Malinowski famously put it, is 'to grasp the native's point of view, his relation to life, to realise *his* vision of *his* world'[5] (which presumably applies to women as well!). Or, as a commitment framed in the first person, 'I want to know what you know *in the way that you know it* . . . will you become my teacher and help me understand?'[6]

A useful aphorism for such a perspective is that 'insight always comes from the inside'. Judgements about whether what is said is true, valid, sensible, real or factual are not such important driving values (as they are in science). The initial assumption, which starts from a different place, is that there is an inherent 'truth-value' in what people say, regardless of whether it actually happened or even happened in the way they say it did ('fact-value'), and it is the (recollected) experienced reality not the 'real reality' (whatever that is) that one is after. For example, Dickens' or Shakespeare's works may be works of fiction yet the insights they give us into the experience of love, loss, and loneliness are no less because they did not actually occur; indeed fiction may sometimes highlight an experience more intensely than the 'real thing'. The books – in our case patient and carer accounts of their treatment experiences – stand up as meaningful and revealing representations of experience in their own right.

Trying to make sense out of how other people make sense

The proper title for the field we are referring to here is *interpretive (or symbolic) anthropology*, which needs to be distinguished from other branches of anthropology which do not have the same interest in the subjective world and the concept of experience. The towering figure in this field is Clifford Geertz (*see* Geertz's classic work, *The Interpretation of Cultures*[7]) who is the leading cultural anthropologist of his generation, and one of the first to focus on the meaning of experience. It was in the 1950s, after a lifetime of conducting ethnographic research within various tribes and societies, that Geertz introduced symbols and cultures into the debate about experience. He pointed out that it is never possible to get at experience directly, but only indirectly through the *meanings* that people – individually and collectively – attach or ascribe to these experiences, meanings that are inscribed in the symbolic structures that they weave around their experience as they struggle to *make sense* of it. In themselves, these are interpretations, and therefore anthropology is really about interpreting other people's interpretations – 'figuring it out':

> *A good interpretation of anything – a poem, a person, a history, a ritual, an institution, a society – takes us into the heart of that of which it is the interpretation. When it does not do that, but leads us instead somewhere else – into an admiration of its own elegance, of its author's cleverness, or of the beauties of Euclidean order – it may have its intrinsic charms, but it is something else than what the task at hand – figuring out what all that rigmarole is about – calls for.*[7]

This makes anthropology essentially a semiotic activity, one that involves *trying to make sense out of how other people make sense*, the incentive being that this holds the key to everything human and social: judgements, attitudes, values, and action. Van Loon recalls Raymond Williams' insight that it is experience that mediates between 'being' and 'consciousness', between that which exists and that which makes sense, thus defining the focus of ethnography as being to 'trace particular instances of sense-making in lived experience'.[8] Not that the task is ever easy, or that you ever truly get to the bottom of it in the form of a 'definitive interpretation', says Geertz:

> *What the ethnographer is in fact faced with ... is a multiplicity of complex conceptual structures, many of them superimposed upon or knotted into one*

another, which are at once strange, irregular, and inexplicit, and which (s)he must contrive somehow first to grasp and then to render . . . Doing ethnography is like trying to read (in the sense of 'construct a reading of') a manuscript – foreign, faded, full of ellipses, incoherencies, suspicious emendations, and tendentious commentaries.[7]

As usual, Geertz is exaggerating somewhat, but this is no bad thing if it succeeds in drawing attention to the fact that figuring out the hieroglyphics of experience is a process that requires enormous patience and skill, and is as far removed from today's focus groups and Discovery Interviews (*see* later) as it could be. To the earlier question, 'what's new?' (Chapter 3) we therefore feel obliged to reply 'almost everything'. Improvement professionals, even those who are listening to and working with narrative and stories, may still not be practising anything that resembles interpretive anthropology, simply because they have not been trained to do so. As Geertz might have put it, barbers may work on heads but that does not make them brain surgeons.

An obvious requirement in trying to figure out and formulate other people's symbol systems is that the endeavour needs to be obsessively other- or (to use the proper phrase) actor-centred. One of the many challenges here is that these other 'actors' will invariably be strangers, and more often than not very different from ourselves by way of background, make-up and present situation. It is never easy to make close contact with the lives of strangers at the best of times, but we have to go still further to remove (more accurately help them to remove) this barrier of strangeness so as to uncover the conceptual structures that inform their acts and experiences.

Doing interpretive anthropology in an improvement design situation involves a variety of activities: engagement, conversation, narration, interpretation, and finally inscription: 'The ethnographer "inscribes" social discourse; *(s)he writes it down*. In so doing, (s)he turns it into an *account*, which exists in its inscriptions and can be reconsulted.'[7] Asking what is the principal thing ethnographers do, Clifford and Marcus thus give the answer, 'They write'.[9]

Thus far, we have traced where the academic interest in 'experience' (in the jargon, 'emic analysis', *see* page 50, or *verstehen*) came from but so far have successfully managed to avoid saying what it actually is! For this we need to go back a step to the broader philosophy of experience which anthropology and the design disciplines use as their source.

The meaning of experience

Experience – that evanescent flux of sensation and perception that is, in some sense, all we have and all we are. (Erik Davis)

The problem of defining 'experience'

Wherever one goes these days, it is hard to avoid having some kind of encounter with 'experience', whether this be the 'ultimate dining experience', 'driving experience', 'fitness experience', 'eBay experience', 'ageing experience', 'holiday experience', 'religious experience' or 'near-death experience'. We even have our very first 'musical experience designer' in the form of ex-Genesis member Peter

Gabriel who has spoken eloquently about involving his audience in designing their own musical experiences:

> *For a number of years I've wanted to become an experience designer rather than just a musician and this new technology is one of the things that is going to allow us to take a step in that direction. Interactivity is exciting because it helps us not just to be artists but to provide a lot of material for the audience to participate in – so that eventually they become artists themselves and can use what we create, in a sense as collage material, as stuff to explore and learn about from the inside.*

If that is confusing, consider what it means today when a yoghurt carton invites you to create your own 'yoghurt experience'. Like most of the other tasty morsels listed here, it sheds not the smallest glimmer of light on what 'experience' is or involves. In fact, the more the term gets popularised, the vaguer and more diluted its meaning seems to become. The problem is not new. There has always been a problem defining experience: 'Experience can mean anything. Experience is rarely defined in a systematic way.'[10]

Phenomenology: the science of experience

So what *is* experience, and what does it mean when we say that we want to understand (grasp or appreciate may be better words) someone else's 'experience' of being a user, consumer or patient – or, as Goffman once rather loftily put it, *the experience of patienthood*?[11] Looking briefly at some of the historical roots of the term will yield some of the answers. 'Experience' has always been a central interest of philosophy, but there is one branch of philosophy that cornered it for its own: (the unattractively titled) 'phenomenology'. (Anthropologists working within this paradigm have even used the term 'phenomenological anthropology' to describe their approach – a phrase almost guaranteed to put anyone off going further to find out what it is!) To put it in context, phenomenology – formally defined as the study of structures of experience – can be distinguished from the four other main fields of philosophy: ontology (the study of being or what is), epistemology (the study of knowledge), logic (the study of reasoning), and ethics (the study of right and wrong).

Martin Heidegger[12,13] and Edmund Husserl,[14] who are credited as being the founding fathers of this 'science of experience', decided that the focus of their new philosophy was to be ordinary, everyday 'lived experience', their aim being to make this accessible, intelligible and, above all, discussable. This idea of studying experience objectively may seem contradictory – is not experience, by its very nature, subjective? Contentiously, Husserl and Heidegger were looking for a rigorous method of describing experience that in fact did away with subjectivity. (Today we would probably be more comfortable with 'representing subjectivity'.) Husserl's motto was 'To the things themselves!' By this he did not mean that he wanted to study things as they exist objectively out there in the world, but rather that he wanted to study the experience of things, as they present themselves to the observer, without any assumptions, predefinitions, interpretations or prejudice as to why or how they exist (or even whether they 'really' exist at all).[15] The attitude is 'I want to understand your world through your eyes and your experiences so far as is possible and together we can probe your experiences fully and understand them.' Their ambition – and that of later contemporaries, famous writers like Jean-Paul Sartre,[16] Maurice Merleau-Ponty[17] and Paul Ricoeur – was to take 'ordinary experience', defined as an ongoing process involving the phenomenal unfolding of awareness in real time[18] – experience as opposed to *an* experience – out of the everyday flow of life (rushing by, unseen, soon forgotten) so as to 'fix' it as a subject and an object of study and analysis (capturing reality in flight). The aim was thus to privilege experience, to make it sort of 'special', to change it from something that was habitual and taken for granted – part of the jetstream of life – to a phenomenon of intrinsic value, curiosity and interest. (We refer readers to Dewey's classic 1930s book *Art as Experience*, especially the chapter 'What is experience?', for further discussion of what constitutes our world of experience.[19])

Thus, rather than being represented as life's cast-off or detritus, experience was recast much more positively by the phenomenologists as sedimentary learning, whose contents – a rich accumulation of previous efforts to solve life's problems, mistakes but also wisdom ('the wisdom of experience') – were seen as holding many of the keys to future designs and solutions. Husserl described the overall endeavour of looking back over experience as returning to the familiar but with a new attitude. The value of this for all of us with an interest in experience is captured in an aphorism that we find ourselves using more and more in our work, that 'hindsight' gives 'insight', and 'insight' gives 'foresight'. Only by reliving our lives backward are we able to live our lives forward – what organisation theorist Karl Weick calls retrospective sense-making, for him the basis of effective learning and action.[20]

Paradoxically, experience may define who we are and what we do and have done, but it is not something we understand that well, or even tend to be that interested in, in our day-to-day lives. This is what makes focusing on it radical – and it *is* a radical idea to really (stress 'really') try to understand the experience of being one of our own children, an immigrant, an adoptive mother, an abused child, drug addict, or dying patient or the dying patient's family (*see* later story on pages 67–8), especially if we have not experienced any of these roles or situations directly for ourselves. The philosophy is 'radical' because it is about heightening awareness (*innewerden*) and insight, and therefore has the potential for being truly transformative – or, as Peter Berger once put it, 'all revolutions begin in transformations of consciousness'. One aspect of the transformative nature of phenomenology is the deep learning about self and others which often occurs from participating in this kind of reflective study.[21] In this context, it is better to begin by acknowledging that you *think* you know, but best to *assume* that you really do not.

The transformative potential of truly accessing someone else's experience is not something that can be demonstrated in the abstract. Rather, readers need to experience first-hand the full force of real examples, which we shall be providing throughout the book (beginning below). Alternatively, they may wish to skip straight to Chapter 9 where they can hear about the kind of things that constitute the experience of being a head and neck cancer patient or their carer. Some of these will not be surprising but others, as we shall show, did come as both a surprise and a revelation, even to those intimately bound up with treating and caring for such patients.

Why understand 'experience' at all?

But first we need to ask: why bother to go to such trouble trying to understand experience? Why not stick with behaviour, which at least is observable, or attitude which is measurable? Simply for the reason that all of our judgements, attitudes, sentiments, feelings, sensations, opinions, memories, actions and reactions are coloured and shaped by our experience, and it is therefore only by understanding, and ultimately designing, experiences that we can influence and begin to understand and create the very 'essence' of life itself. Nevertheless, the task is far from easy or straightforward, since experience has many of the characteristics of the will o' the wisp, that largely invisible and mischievous spirit of a dead life. The core problem in studying experience is that, as an 'inner' subjective, immaterial phenomenon, it can never be accessed or observed directly, only indirectly through the words and language people use to describe it when they look back over it and try to describe and recall it. In this sense it is not 'real' at all (as it actually was or is at the time) but a reconstruction or reconstitution of something lived through and now passed – an elapsed, recalled experience. Words put meaning on that experience reflectively and retrospectively, and represent 'what I make of what I have lived through'. As radical activist Saul Alinsky once so nicely put it:

> *Happenings become experiences when they are digested, when they are reflected on, related to general patterns and synthesised.*[22]

Words are the vessels or messengers of meaning and experience, capable of transporting an unanalysable past into an analysable present in the form of stories and anecdotes. This is why narrative and storytelling play such an important part in EBD's armoury of methods, in fact are indispensable to its practice (*see* Chapter 6). As the first of many real-life examples in this book we invite the reader to consider how the words in the following story convey the experiences of a father – who happens to be a GP (general practitioner) – coming to terms with his 16-year-old daughter's mental illness:

> *We thought it was a typical school thing, being bullied and we just thought we'd got a very difficult child. I had a General Practice; my wife's a district nurse and we just sailed into it looking for a good life really. We decided it was a good job, really nice place to work; it was good, it was easy. We got all sorted out, middle-class and it was all going very well and then something happens. So [my daughter] became difficult and I thought that was about the worst adolescence I'd seen. I'd been going to lots of families as a GP, quite dysfunctional families and in our own family things seemed far worse; I couldn't understand why. That was odd and then she started to see faces at the window and stuff and we began to realise that things weren't right and then she tried to kill herself. She put some paper into a socket; she brought us upstairs to see her do it and we suddenly thought, 'God, this is something serious.'*
>
> *At that point we sort of panicked, probably appropriately. So we called in for help. A psychiatrist comes in from a children's service and does a domiciliary at home and says [my daughter's] got schizophrenia. And we were surprised because [my wife] had done psychiatric nursing and hadn't seen it. We thought she was depressed and was being bullied . . . Then we had a fascinating*

12 months with nice people, good staff . . . but they've got no services. So essentially we had a two-weekly appearance at a grotty little children's outpatients. Kids' toys . . . You know for a 16-year-old and the toys are Teletubbies or something and you're sat there thinking you're not in the right place and it was grotty. And the psychiatrist, God bless him, used to say, 'There's nothing we can offer here. We don't' – I think his words were – 'if you just hang on to the adult service then we're into psychosis', and for 12 months you had nothing more than that.

So eventually there was a bank holiday weekend, Mothering Sunday actually, and I was on call. It was my 30th phone call and [my daughter] was convinced that every phone call was about her and we just couldn't contain it; she became very angry, very distressed, running around the house. We had 12 months and that was it really. She had a paranoia extended to not just me, because that was one of the difficulties, very, very paranoid towards me, but when that paranoia extended to mum and grandma, who's a key figure, that's it, it just fell apart. So within 48 hours she found herself in an acute adult ward so, at just 17, into the most chaotic environment you could ever believe. It was bedlam really. And for 48 hours of that we thought, it was the first time we'd ever had a break really for 12 months. [My wife] had given up her job. I was lucky to go out to work and that was it. So we thought, 48 hours, wow – we can just relax.

And there's two other kids in this family and there is us and then we realised that first of all [my daughter's] illness was getting worse in this environment – it was such a punitive and inappropriate environment really – and she spent six months in an acute adult ward because there was nowhere else for a 17-year-old with a psychosis to go. I was told it was that rare, but you know, it was not that rare. Everyone told us it would get slightly better, but it all seemed to get worse and when anyone made a prediction it didn't improve, it got worse. So we realised that we were in a service that didn't deal with young people. We'd gone from a children's service that didn't do psychosis to an adult centre that didn't do young people. It was daft. I couldn't have dreamt of designing a service that was more inappropriate for teenage onset of this psychosis, this 15 to 25-ish age group.

So six months there. Eventually it was suggested that she go into a rehab setting and that was in the old 'bin' where I was a GP and practised there. And there was this asylum and I used to drive past it and used to be GP to quite a few of the staff and I never understood it really. And then I did understand it. This rehab was a lie – it wasn't rehab at all really; it was just a warehouse, eight-bedded dormitory, no carpets, no curtains, $17^1/_2$ years old, going nowhere really. It was always getting worse.

Then there was a transformative incident which was Jane. Jane arrived as a new psychiatrist and within three or four days of her being in post, literally within days, she called [my wife] and I to her office and said she thinks she'll complain. So that was a transformational moment. And Jane explained that there wasn't things, like there wasn't an OT [occupational therapist], there wasn't a psychologist. She said she would deal with that but she's just a psychiatrist and she was being quite blunt about what the service didn't have. And she also said that [my daughter] had got a very bad illness and they would do their best, but you know . . . I think the real basis of that point was, how can this be right for a 16 ¹/₂, 17-year-old, putting her into a bin with no possible hope – it is totally hopeless – and the only thing you thought would be crazy was some sort of monster. There was never going to be anything of a life; she was just blighted really and that's how it would be. And her future was mapped out – she was going to stay in an institution for the rest of her days and our shoulders would be down as a family. It felt very, very grey – not so much angry as very grey. I couldn't see any future. I just craved for the boys to leave home and find a future and [my wife] and I would just be doomed – this is your path. And I couldn't see any way out of it. So, in a sense, all we did was go from day to day. [My wife] and I used to talk at night when the kids were asleep and just say, well, that's another day. Deep down, I think, I was very, very distressed.

At this point we do not wish to say anything that may detract from this illustration of the sheer power of narrative to convey experience in the raw. Analysis will come later, and will need to if narrative and experience are to be connected up to design, but for the moment that can wait. And of course this is just one perspective, the experience of a father; now add to that the experience of the daughter herself, his wife, Jane and others, and we begin to see how multilayered, nuanced, and therefore frighteningly complex experience is. On the other hand, just reflect on the amount of knowledge and wisdom that resides unused in such a bundle of stories, and why it is therefore imperative to find some way of harnessing it in the service design activity.

Elements of experience

We turn now to the various elements that make up experience. Writers differentiate between various 'forms of experience' (which collectively define the phenomenon), and suggest that all of them have a place in 'phenomenological anthropology'. The idiomatic term for these forms is the 'look-and-feel' or 'think–feel–do' factors (see Garrett's seminal graphic[23]) – the head, heart and hand – but more specifically (and here it might be worth thinking back to the above story using these categories) they include:

- reflection and awareness (of self, others, environment, time, space – initially the conscious stuff at the centre of attention, but then moving to the periphery of attention where people are only vaguely aware of things)
- sensation (kinesthetics: sight, hearing, touch, etc., in terms of degree of pleasantness)
- perception (as in seeing a sunset, or hearing birdsong)
- thought (thinking about love, illness, pain)
- memory (remembering care and kindness)
- imagination (a safe, peaceful world)
- emotion and expression (feeling fear, anxiety, pleasure and happiness)
- desire (wanting something or someone)
- volition (intending to acquire or achieve something)
- action and conduct (bungee jumping!).

It is clear from this list that there is considerably more to experience than 'look-and-feel', and this is exactly what Fulton Suri is getting at when she says that 'designers are being invited to influence not just the look and feel of individual things, but the quality of experience that people have as they live their lives through time and space'.[24] Healthcare designers also need to pay heed to this, their task being the broader one of improving the whole quality of experience and not settling for changing the look and feel of, say, a front entrance or clinic.

Norman and colleagues help us to get closer to the materials from which the 'quality of experience' is fashioned.[25] These include:

- *affect*: what a person feels, the affective quality of an experience, for example one's emotional response to a diagnosis or treatment
- *motivation/value*: how the experience is seen in cost–benefit terms as adding value at a psychological or economic level, for example a mastectomy which is known to save one's life but has a negative effect on one's self-image or feelings about oneself; the idea of experience as net value
- *cognition*: what the person, knows, thinks and believes in relation to a care or treatment episode.

The brief statements below describing a visit to a hospital illustrate just how these many facets of experience might reveal themselves.

A visit to the hospital: 'my experience'

'I am aware *my heart is beating quickly, and I am starting to sweat; other patients seem less anxious than I am; I am aware of a stony silence within the waiting room.' (affect)*

'I get this strong sense *of feeling exposed and vulnerable in this strange environment.' (affect)*

'I see *the trolleys of very sick people coming and going, and catch those char-acteristic smells of a hospital: disinfectant, cabbage, smoke.' (cognition)*

'I think *what am I doing here and is it too late to run?' (motivation/value)*

'I remember *something my GP said . . .' (cognition)*

'I consider *is the pain worth the gain? (motivation/value)*

'I imagine *getting out of here as quickly as possible.' (cognition)*

'I am feeling *incredibly tired, and my limbs are heavy.' (affect)*

'I would love *a nice cup of tea, and a kind word from someone.' (affect)*

'I intend *telling the doctor something I have never told anyone before.' (cognition)*

'So now I have to decide*: am I going to carry on living with the pain or lose some of the mobility in my limb?' (net value)*

Collectively these make up a person's *reality-as-experienced*,[26] which is not only what phenomenology is interested in but also what one is trying to get at in the early stages of design.

The challenge of experience-based design

Reflecting on other kinds of experience – especially intense ones of the raw, adrenalin-rush variety, like riding on a rollercoaster, engaging in extreme sports, going to a rock concert, undergoing a spiritual or religious conversion, or falling in love – is another way of getting a grasp of what experience is all about, and why it is so important to all of us. The challenge for the researcher and designer, however, is to be able to help the storyteller go beyond bland statements like 'that was great' or 'that was really scary', and find the words to convey how it *was* for them. Therein lies the challenge of EBD, of being able to progress from sharing an experience to deriving concrete *knowledge* about how that experience might be improved the next time one finds oneself in that situation.

The broad approach phenomenologists recommend for anyone trying to understand another person's experience is that the listener needs to *try* to suspend all 'contaminating presuppositions' he or she may have about what it means, or must mean/feel like for the interviewee or teller. 'Try' is the active word. Most anthropologists today would accept that this is no more than an aspiration, a way of opening up the channels and receptors to the participant's 'life-view'. Empathy is the key; and here we are talking about empathy as both technique and frame of mind. The *technique* of empathy involves consciously taking on the role or mantle of the stranger, the innocent, the person who readily acknowledges that she herself has not had the same experiences as, say, the patient being interviewed, cannot know what it was really like, and may need to ask some pretty dumb questions of someone who clearly does. Maso draws on Alfred Schutz's classic, part-autobiographical essay on 'the stranger' to suggest how by deliberately casting ourselves as outsiders to this experience, and professing ignorance of the insider's ways, we trigger an interaction and discovery process in which we are taught what it means to experience being (say) a patient in this situation.[27]

The Japanese have the phrase 'sen sei' which translates as 'in front of . . . students'. The idea is that someone, in this case the teacher, 'has knowledge' someone else does not have. This fits nicely with the idea that experience is knowledge that needs to be taught; however, unlike the Japanese example, it is the patient who has the 'sen sei' who is the teacher, and the experience researcher the pupil. Therefore, in an interesting role reversal, the patient becomes the expert, the instructor or educator, mentor to you the mentee, master to apprentice. No longer are they your 'subject'. They are now the main characters in the play and you are their understudy. Still one of the best elaborations of the novice or 'sorcerer's apprentice' role is Carlos Castaneda's cult book series of the 1970s and 1980s in which he, the green-horn UCLA PhD student, meets and strikes up an unlikely friendship with Don Juan, a Mexican Yaqui Indian who becomes his teacher and then proceeds to introduce him to his 'life world', involving experiences that are entirely, and often frighteningly, alien from his own.[28] Garfinkel described the researcher's role similarly as being that of a 'secret apprentice'.[29] In many ways, Castaneda is still the best role model for today's experience researcher, a courageous, humble individual who was prepared to suspend disbelief, listen deeply and learn, and although there is inequality in his relationship with his teacher, there is also loyalty, love and respect.

This is the point at which the anthropological method of participant observation begins to come in to play: *participant* because it is only by working among and close to one's subjects (co-collaborator or co-participant is obviously better), and, by degrees, gaining access to their 'symbolic life world' that one can ascertain the inner subjective logic on which it is built, and feel, hear and see a little of life as one's 'subjects' do. But also as *observer* one is deliberately standing back, taking the outside-insider position of the cultural foreigner or stranger in order to see and ask questions that may appear irrelevant, strange or pointless from your subject's point of view. This is where the idea of 'affected naivety' comes in:

> *The ethnographer must in this sense be sometimes a little naïve by design – becoming the outsider who does not quite understand what is going on, asking for information which everyone either knows already or does not wish to probe.*[30]

The general idea is that the more I, the experience researcher, engage, question and help people to reflect on their experiences from this outside-inside position, *the more I shall be able to imagine myself in these experiences*, and the more I become able understand them. So, first, I have to help them to get in touch with their own experiences, and second, they have to help me to get in touch with their experiences (subjectivity). Finally, what we have to do together is cross-check, and keep cross-checking, these recollections and interpretations for veracity and authenticity against the original experience (inter-subjectivity). Of course, they will always be approximations of the real experience, even for the patients themselves:

> *There is no way of seeing, hearing or representing the world of others that is absolutely, universally valid or correct. Ethnographies of any sort are always subject to multiple interpretations. They are never beyond controversy or debate.*[31]

Arguably, and ironically, arrived at inter-subjectively they may still be closer to the reality than could ever be achieved through objective scientific methods.

Much of the success of the joint reflective process described here depends on the quality of the relationship that is established, and in this regard Powdermaker is absolutely right when she describes the way of an anthropologist as 'stranger and friend',[32] as is Clifford Geertz when he talks about having 'close-in contact with far-out lives'.[33] 'Friend' implies confidence, fidelity and trust, and a feeling – knowledge – that they are on your side and will not exploit any disclosures you choose to make about yourself. EBD without this quality of relationship will not succeed, which is why so much effort has to go into building and proving that relationship between all those involved, especially in the early stages of the process. In this sense 'building the change relationship' is as important in EBD as it is in any other form of organisational development.

References

1 Experience Designer Network. Design. What is experience design? www.experi-encedesignernetwork.com/archives/00368.html (accessed 2 August 2006).
2 Bate SP. Whatever happened to organisational anthropology? A review of the field of organisational ethnography and anthropological studies. *Human Relations.* 1997; **50**(9): 1147–75.
3 Gephart RP. Qualitative research and the Academy of Management Journal. *Academy of Management Journal.* 2004; **47**(4): 454–62.
4 Schein EH. Vita contemplative. From brainwashing to organisational therapy: a conceptual and empirical journey in search of 'systemic' health and a general model of change dynamics. A drama in five acts. *Organisation Studies.* 2006; **27**(2): 287–301.
5 Malinowski B. *Argonauts of the Western Pacific: An Account of Native Enterprise and Adventure in the Archipelagos of Melanesian New Guinea.* London: Routledge & Kegan Paul; 1922.

6 Spradley JP. *The Ethnographic Interview.* Orlando, FL: Harcourt Brace Jovanovich; 1979.

7 Geertz C. *The Interpretation of Cultures.* New York: Basic Books; 1973.

8 Van Loon J. Ethnography: a critical turn in cultural studies. In: Atkinson P, Coffey A, Delamont S *et al.*, editors. *Handbook of Ethnography.* London: Sage; 2001. p. 273–84.

9 Clifford J, Marcus GE. *Writing Culture. The Poetics and Politics of Ethnography.* Berkeley, CA: California University Press; 1986.

10 Skeggs B. Feminist ethnography. In: Atkinson P, Coffey A, Delamont S *et al.*, editors. *Handbook of Ethnography.* London: Sage; 2001. p. 426–42.

11 Goffman E. *Asylums: Essays on the Social Situation of Mental Patients and Other Inmates.* New York: Doubleday Anchor; 1961.

12 Heidegger M. *Being and Time.* (Macquarrie J, Robinson E, trans.) New York: Harper & Row; 1962 (first edition 1927).

13 Heidegger M. *Poetry, Language and Thought.* New York; Harper & Row; 1971.

14 Husserl E. *Ideas: A General Introduction in Pure Phenomenology.* (Boyce Gibson WR, trans., original 1913.) New York: Collier Books; 1963.

15 Kissell J. Phenomenonology. The science of experience. 6 July 2004. http://itotd.com/index.alt?ArticleID=237 (accessed 2 August 2006).

16 Sartre J-P. *Being and Nothingness.* (Barnes H, trans., original 1943.) New York: Washington Square Press; 1956.

17 Merleau-Ponty M. *Phenomenology of Perception.* (Smith C, trans., original 1945.) New York: Routledge; 1996.

18 Davis E. Experience design and the design of experience. 2000. www.techgnosis.com/experience.html (accessed 2 August 2006).

19 Dewey J. Art as experience. In: Boydston JA, series editor. *John Dewey: The Later Works, 1925–1953, Vol. 10: 1934.* Carbondale: Southern Illinois University Press; 1987.

20 Weick KE. *Making Sense of the Organisation.* Oxford: Blackwell; 2001.

21 Perl EJ. Phenomenology: transforming research and practice. *Passages.* 1996; Winter.

22 Alinsky SD. *Rules for Radicals. A Pragmatic Primer for Realistic Radicals.* New York: Vintage Books; 1972.

23 Garrett JJ. *The Elements of User Experience, User-Centred Design for the Web.* Berkeley, CA: New Riders Publishing; 2002.

24 Fulton Suri J. Empathetic design: informed and inspired by other people's experience. In: Koskinen I, Batterbee K, Mattelmaki T, editors. *Empathetic Design – User Experience in Product Design.* Helsinki: IT Press; 2003. p. 51–8.

25 Norman DA, Ortony A, Revelle W. Effective functioning: a three level model of affect, behaviour and cognition. In: Fellous JM, Arbib MA, editors. *Who Needs Emotions? The Brain Meets the Machine.* New York: Oxford University Press; 2005.

26 Harper D. *Working Knowledge: Skill and Community in a Small Shop.* Berkeley, CA: University of California Press; 1992.

27 Maso I. Phenomenology and ethnography. In: Atkinson P, Coffey A, Delamont S *et al.*, editors. *Handbook of Ethnography.* London: Sage; 2001. p. 136–44.

28 Castaneda C. *The Teachings of Don Juan: A Yaqui Way of Knowledge.* New York: Washington Square Press; 1985.

29 Garfinkel H. *Studies in Ethnomethodology.* Englewood Cliffs, NJ: Prentice-Hall; 1967.

30 Rock P. Symbolic interaction and ethnography. In: Atkinson P, Coffey A, Delamont S *et al.*, editors. *Handbook of Ethnography.* London: Sage; 2001. p. 26–38.

31 Van Maanen J. *Tales of the Field. On Writing Ethnography.* Chicago: The University of Chicago Press; 1988.

32 Powdermaker H. *Stranger and Friend: The Way of an Anthropologist.* New York: WW Norton; 1966.

33 Geertz C. *Work and Lives. The Anthropologist as Author.* Cambridge: Polity Press; 1988.

Part 2

Methods

Having discussed the concepts of 'design' and 'experience' in the first part of this book, our second part (Chapters 5–8) is concerned with the methods that accompany the EBD process. The section begins by detailing the basic disciplinary principles and features that underpin an EBD approach (Chapter 5). The chapter details four guiding principles for those interested in exploring 'experience': the need for immersion, the need for openness, the need for rigour and the need for empathy. The next chapter places particular emphasis on exploring further the importance – and analysis – of stories and storytelling (Chapter 6). Chapter 7 then introduces the notion of 'patterns-based design' (encompassing patterns and anti-patterns), using two examples (the 'immediate feedback' principle – including the importance of 'entry' and 'exit' experiences – and the rule of progressive disclosure). Chapter 8 then explores a wide range of specific methods and techniques for (a) *diagnosing* user experiences, and (b) *making an intervention* to improve user experiences. This chapter then concludes with a brief retelling of a case study that explores how redesigning physical environments can be successfully combined with efforts to redesign experience.

Chapter 5

Becoming a disciple of experience

*The rules of experience are all that is needed to discern the true from the false;
experience is what helps all men to look temperately for the possible, rather
than cloaking oneself in ignorance, which can result in no good thing,
so that, in the end, one abandons oneself to despair and melancholy.*
(Leonardo da Vinci)

Leonardo da Vinci once famously described himself as a 'disciple of experience',
claiming experience to be his mistress, his one true muse, the one thing that
allowed him to paint, write or invent despite his lack of formal education or academic training. So what was he getting at, and how does one become a 'disciple
of experience' in a modern-day organisational context – and why bother?
Recapping on what has already been said, it seems the only way the disciple can
get his or her spurs is by engaging in both (a) description, and (b) interpretation
(of experience). These two broad requirements may be broken down further to
include the following.

- Making someone else's personal experience(s) (the raw data of phenomenological study) the object and focus of attention; in other words, becoming
  'mindful' of experience from the first-person point of view, in our case usually the 'customer's':

  *Fundamental to any effort is understanding experience from the customer's
  perspective – that is, seeing what the customer sees, hearing what the customer
  hears, touching what the customer touches, smelling what the customer smells,
  tasting what the customer tastes, and, above all, feeling what the customer feels.
  Organisations need to work to become more clue conscious and understand the
  level of subtle details that are processed in customers' conscious and unconscious thoughts impacting how they feel in an experience.*[1]

- Engaging with them in explicit 'retrospection', 'recapitulation' and 'reflexive
  awareness' (what Alfred Schutz summed up as 'the reflective glance').
- Producing some kind of mental construct map of that experience (hence our
  later term, 'experience mapping', which is about the person and the (internal) experience they went through, as opposed to 'process mapping', which
  is about the (external) system or process their care passed through), which
  will ultimately show both real and ideal experiences alongside each other (*see*
  Figure 9.3 on page 139).
- Enabling that experience to be retrieved, interpreted, abstracted and made
  meaningful, i.e. the 'sense' we now make of what we lived through (sense-
  making always being retrospective).
- In re-living that experience, making it 'mine', and in sharing it, making it
  'ours' (the important issue of ownership and commitment in change and
  improvement).

Four principles for disciples (and a fifth: some fun)

There are four principles related to these requirements that need to be carefully attended to by budding experience disciples.

The first principle is that of *immersion*. The word 'immersion' crops up a good deal in anthropology and phenomenology, and figures prominently in the work of scholars like Erving Goffman, Robert Park and Howard Becker. Goffman honoured deep immersion and would ultimately have the fieldworker acquire the rhythms and personal aesthetics of those studied. This does not mean having to go the whole hog like some erstwhile overzealous anthropologists have done in the past by taking psychotropic medication in order to have the experience of former mental patients, or spending three years training to be a boxer in order to experience and convey the 'passion, love and suffering' of being in the sport![2] However, it is generally recognised that, while brain damage is not essential to the endeavour, ethnographers do still need to go fairly deep into experience itself in order to make an interpretive rendering – the notion of *immersive understanding*.

As Bergson puts it, there are two ways of knowing a thing.[3] The first is going all around it, the second entering into it – as if visiting a place. The ethnographer's job is to explore the second way. The corollary to this principle is that, as one does this, it is important to remain stubbornly experience-focused from the beginning,[4] as opposed to attitude-, systems- or process-focused. Modern design companies like IDEO (www.ideo.com) talk about taking 'deep dives' into experience, and the metaphor is a useful one because of the implication that one needs to strive to go deeper than 'surface' attitudes, holding one's breath for as long as one can (i.e. suspending judgement). For examples of healthcare interventions involving deep dives (Memorial Hospital in the US being one), readers should visit: www.ideo.com/portfolio/re.asp?x=50185 (accessed 3 August 2006). Such ethnographic methods as we are describing here, i.e. actor-centred, polyphonic or multivocal, consist of 'thick description', and naturally lead back to immersion. The British philosopher Gilbert Ryle's (cited by Geertz[5]) notion of 'thick description' is what you would expect from the name – rich, close-to accounts of events and activities, as opposed to the parsimonious radically thinned descriptions of science – but beyond this it also includes the ability to distinguish between things which appear to be identical (and where the difference is unphotographable) but are not; for example a twitch or a wink, or even a fake-wink, all visibly the same but meaning something entirely different. Thick description is therefore the ability to say with some degree of certainty not only what a person is doing and what is happening (behaviourism) but what that something actually means to the person doing it (interpretation). Although today, through necessity, a lot of this ethnography in an organisational context is of the 'quick and dirty' variety,[6] quick description rather than thick description,[7] much of its unique value will be lost if it abandons this commitment to interpretation and experience entirely.

The second guiding principle is never to make assumptions that you *know* what someone else's experience is, or that it is anything like how you might experience it for yourself. It is not the outsider's role to test hypotheses (which assumes you do know something already) but rather to let the user lead the interaction (i.e. the old OD (organisational development) rules of 'start with the client' and it being safer to assume you probably don't know anything about what it is really like). The key here is to focus on the central, dominant or recurring themes which represent the essential qualities or meanings of the participant's experience (called thematisation and structuring). It is important not to use a theoretical model to access experience, at least not in the first instance. Instead, one should try to be a-theoretical or pre-theoretical and 'open' and 'grounded' in the life world of the subject.

The correct label for this kind of approach is 'emic', meaning viewed from the actor's point of view, rather than the 'etic' outside observer or non-participant viewpoint. The neologisms 'emic' and 'etic', which were derived from an analogy with the terms 'phonemic' and 'phonetic', were coined by the linguistic anthropologist Kenneth Pike,[8] who suggested that there are two perspectives that can be employed in the study of a society's cultural system, just as there are two perspectives that can be used in the study of a language's sound system. In both cases, it is possible to take the point of view of either the insider or the outsider. As Pike defines it, the emic perspective focuses on the intrinsic cultural distinctions that are meaningful to the members of a given society themselves (for example, whether the natural world is distinguished from the supernatural realm in the worldview of the culture) in the same way that phonemic analysis focuses on the intrinsic phonological distinctions that are meaningful to speakers of a given language. The etic perspective, again according to Pike, relies upon the extrinsic concepts and categories that have meaning for scientific observers (for example, per capita energy consumption) in the same way that phonetic analysis relies upon the extrinsic concepts and categories that are meaningful to linguistic analysts (for example, dental fricatives). Scientists are the sole judges of the validity of an etic account, just as linguists are the sole judges of the accuracy of a phonetic transcription.

Consequently, explorative co-experiences should not and can not be planned in any detail in advance (this being different from preparation, which can and should take place); they happen because a possibility has presented itself at a suitable moment. Such interactions are therefore characterised by flexibility, emergence and opportunism. As Van Maanen confesses:

> *Accident and happenstance shapes fieldworkers' studies as much as planning or foresight; numbing routine as much as living theatre; impulse as much as rational choice; mistaken judgements as much as accurate ones. This may not be the way fieldwork is reported, but it is the way it is done.*[9]

Design research, like most qualitative research, is often designed at the same time it is being done, and requires highly contextualised individual judgements (for more detail on this see Van Maanen[10]). The flowing 'ongoing consciousness' that drives – or should drive – EBD is different from organised experiences such as parties, which are planned beforehand, sometimes down to the smallest detail.[11] In an organisational setting, where there is often a strong cultural preference or requirement for this kind of detailed planning – and often motivated by the same desire or need to reduce anxiety about the uncertainty of what may happen – the required 'hang loose' mentality, and a high tolerance for ambiguity may present a major challenge to some staff members (although in our experience less so for patients).

What might help is to appreciate that there is nothing sloppy or 'unmanagerial' in this: experience flows between the states of subconscious, cognitive, narrative and storytelling[12] and it is impossible to predict, even less to control, the direction this will take, hence the need to be aware of where you are at any time, and to use all your native skills to manage where you came from and are going to. The skill of the EBD facilitator lies not just in the ability to find a way through to experience, but also in his or her ability to 'unfreeze' or enable this expressive process to begin, finding the thermals and positive feedback loops that allow it to gather energy, expand and develop – another managerial skill.

Thus we come to the third principle which is to be no less rigorous and systematic in your endeavours than any scientist would be; to be aware of your own biases, everyday understandings, beliefs and judgements and then shelve or suspend them as best you can.

The fourth and final principle is to listen (with respect) and empathise – or as Lauer puts it so wonderfully, 'experiencing the experiences of others is called empathy';[13] this means coming as close as you can to understanding the experiences being lived by the participants as they do, which involves you 'mentally putting yourself in their place'[14] while at the same time opening up and sharing your own experience and 'take' on what is being said. Informality, participation, collaboration and empathy are therefore the watchwords for this aspect of EBD.[15] Battarbee coins the word 'co-experience' to draw attention to the fact that EBD is not only about experience as something private and individual but, as soon as it begins to be shared in a co-design process, becomes social and public as well.[11] Clinicians and designers involved in co-design have often told us of their surprise in discovering, from what is often their first experience of meaningful social interaction with their patients (meaning- as distinct from information-exchange) just how different their patients' worldviews and perceptions were from their own in relation to the service they were providing (*see* Chapter 9 for some examples from the case study). Such surprise is a sure sign of successful immersion and empathy.

A summary of the phenomenological method – eating ice cream and what makes a cup a cup

The meaning of an experience is recovered and re-enacted in a host of different ways, for example in remembrance, narration, meditation, or more systematically – and this is where the philosophy and discipline come in – through phenomenological interpretation and 'inscription'.[16] The details of the phenomenological method have been described in the following formal, but down-to-earth, manner which, as we can see, incorporates most of the principles described above:

> *It is involved and time-consuming. The first step is to consider the memory of a recent experience – phenomenology is not normally done in real time – and subject it to a process known variously as epoché, bracketing, or phenomenological reduction. Much like the Cartesian method of doubt, epoché [from the Greek meaning 'abstention'] is a temporary suspension of any external beliefs, placing one's focus on the 'raw' experience itself. The goal is to ignore empirical data – along with intuitions and judgements – and simply describe your experience in detail. To take a fairly trivial example, a phenomenological description of eating ice cream would not include a list of ingredients, information about fat or calories, or the likely impact on one's waistline. Instead, the description*

> *includes details about the flavour, temperature, texture, colour, and so on. In other words, you don't concern yourself with what appears, but rather, with a thing's way of appearing.*
>
> *After this, you perform a further process known as eidetic reduction. This involves taking certain features of the bracketed experience and imagining variations on them, as freely as you can. For example, if I am focusing on how a cup appears to me, I may perform free variation on the feature colour, changing it to different hues, or attempting to remove the feature completely. The purpose of this exercise is to arrive at the features that are essential to the object in question. Thus I should discover, for example, that while no one particular colour is essential to a cup's being a cup, it is essential that it have some colour. This is an essential feature of a cup in my experience.*[17]

Though the examples given here are far removed from the world of health and healthcare design, the basic method and sequence of recalling–describing–bracketing–imagining–varying are very much the same as would be used in making sense of – and then taking the next step of acting to improve – a particular experience of healthcare.

. . . and the important fifth principle

There is one final principle to consider in regard to the design approach, namely that the process should be as playful as possible – an exercise in 'funology',[18,19] exploratory, improvisatory, creative, iterative, even childish in nature.[18] Typically, the methods used will therefore tend to be low-tech (often including methods adapted from the children's classroom,[20,21] i.e. lots of cardboard and scissors![22]). Here we are not talking about something that is a luxury but a necessity. The reason lies in the artistic nature of the endeavour which requires all of these qualities of process. Dewey stated that experience created by people interacting (as happens in the EBD process) is closer to art and drama than to sociology and psychology.[23] In other words, it involves creativity and interaction, and lots of serious fun. As the architect Frank Gehry notes in the following, the free flowing fun part ('free play idea'), which in the organisation literature is sometimes referred to as 'institutionalised foolishness', can be found in both art and science, and, reiterating Dewey, is fundamental to creativity and innovation breakthroughs:

> *When the artists and sculptors I know work, there's a sort of free play idea. You try things; you experiment. It's kind of naïve and childish, it's like kids in a playpen. Scientists work that way too – for example, genetic scientists that I have been involved with seem to work similarly. It's kind of like throwing things out and then following the idea, rather than predicting where you're going to go.*[24]

Similarly putting the case for fun and enjoyment in design, Monk and colleagues write that 'we need to refocus our research interests from the negative "stressors" to the positive "motivators"'.[25] The comment is interesting because it has clear resonances with the contemporary literature of OD and change management which has been advocating a major shift from the traditional 'deficiency-based', problem-centred approaches to change to an approach that is altogether more upbeat, energised, ambitious and optimistic, such as Appreciative Inquiry[26] which seeks to concentrate on bringing out the best of the human condition. The equivalent in sociology, psychology and organisation studies has been 'Positive (Organisational) Scholarship' (POS) which broadly states that progress in any domain is likely to be greater, and creative breakthroughs more likely to occur, if we start from the position that the glass is half full rather than half empty.[27] By approaching all human endeavours, including design, from the positive view-point of creating a product or service that is exceptional, virtuous, and life-giving, rather than merely a solution to a need or problem, we are more likely to produce something (including a healthcare system) that enhances the quality of life and not just solves the problem. A service design process that feels more like leisure than work, that is more game-like and playful, and that focuses on fun and enjoyment rather than routine tasks, is more likely to generate energy, creativity and vigilance against mediocrity.[25,28]

At this point we would not wish to overemphasise the differences that people may find between traditional 'process mapping' in healthcare (which is rooted in the 'science of improvement') and 'experience mapping' (rooted in a design approach that combines art, science and drama) – after all the former does use low-tech tools such as brown wallpaper and lots of post-its to map the process in a fun way. However, we would still note in passing that EBD, in our experience, starts with the somewhat different intent of avoiding the 'problems' on which process mapping focuses (such as bottlenecks and phases in the process that do not add value) and looking instead for opportunities and solutions. EBD concentrates upon how a process 'feels' rather than how it 'is'; avoiding what social psychologists call the limits of 'cognitive rationality' (reasoning, logic and depersonalisation of issues) and, in so doing, allowing – encouraging – emotionality and personal involvement to shine through; constantly striving to combine reason with passion, functionality with aesthetics, creativity with analysis, science with art. Again, rather than deal with this discussion in the abstract, readers might prefer to turn at this point to Chapter 9, and judge for themselves whether the EBD process described does indeed feel different to them with respect to the features outlined here.

As we have already pointed out, a number of the EBD principles described in the above have their origins in ethnography and ethnographic methods, and it is therefore perhaps wise to stay as close to these origins as one possibly can. So to recap briefly, the spirit of 'ethnography' is one of 'learning by going' (Geertz), not overly planning but pitching in and 'getting one's hands dirty',[29] the broad methodological challenge being to 'penetrate another form of life' (some feel to be penetrated by is more accurate), to capture the richness of experience, and above all, to grasp 'the "native's" point of view'. As already indicated, a variety of methods may be employed to this end, including narrative and storytelling (*see* Chapter 6 for more detailed discussion), attending meetings and events, documentary investigation of records, and participant observation.[7] These are covered in detail in Chapter 8.

'Action anthropology'

Doing ethnography in a design or action research setting – 'action ethnography'[30,31] – is a more recent development, however, in which the anthropologist becomes co-designer and change agent and anthropological data is fed back to participants to be used in the change/improvement process itself. (For a wider discussion of the idea of doing ethnography in an organisation development or action research setting *see* Bate[30] and Bate and Robert.[32] Chapter 9 of this book also details how an ethnographic approach can contribute to EBD in a healthcare setting.)

In the modern world of 'action-based anthropology', which would be completely alien to Geertz and his academic generation, there is one further step to the interpretive process, namely interacting with, and feeding back that reading or account to, the original owner, and agreeing – or, more accurately, jointly validating – its veracity, authenticity and plausibility. (One wonders how the natives themselves would have reacted to Geertz's famous interpretation of a Balinese cockfight, Malinowski's interpretation of the *kula* of the Trobrianders, or Margaret Mead's reading of the sex lives of South Sea Islanders. Badly, one suspects.) Although today's practising action ethnographers (a combination of analyst and change agent) have their interpretations much more exposed to the acid test of the customer, they do have the advantage over the traditional anthropologist because they are not interacting with dead runes trying to figure it all out for themselves, but talking to the very people that chiselled the words in the first place, getting it from the horse's mouth as it were, checking it out and trying to establish their 'real' meaning and significance *with them*. This is why interpretive anthropology in action settings needs to be not only actor-centred but also highly interactive, so as to provide adequate opportunities for reciprocal reflection, sense-making and learning to occur.

Traditional anthropology cannot escape criticism on this 'action' front, for, as Bloor[33] states in her extensive and thoughtful critique of the literature, while there have been some wonderful ethnographic studies of health and medicine – including classics such as Erving Goffman's *Asylums,*[34] Anselm Strauss and colleagues' *Social Organization of Medical Work,*[35] Roth's *Timetables* (a study of tuberculosis patients)[36] and Howard Becker and colleagues' *Boys in White*[37] – 'medical ethnographies . . . remain highly marginal to clinical practice' (and, we might add, healthcare policy). Have healthcare anthropologists made a difference to the quality of care? Probably not. Rather they have remained timid, not to say sniffy, about getting too close to the action, their fear apparently being the loss of that highly prized quality of 'critical detachment'. Within a design sciences frame, however, all this changes – indeed has to change. The anthropologists are required to come down from their perch and engage in real-life human interaction, no longer observing from afar (a more unkind word would be 'voyeurism') but participating and seeking to influence and impact on the world around them.

We shall describe this use of ethnographic data as an intervention in the case study in Chapter 9 but an important component of such an approach (which is explicitly designed to 'make a difference') draws on another stream of design thinking: participatory design.

Participatory design + experience design = experience-based co-design

Adherence to the features and principles listed earlier in this chapter leads one naturally to an experience-based co-design approach, which is actually a confluence of two streams of design thinking: participatory design and experience design (which – as we have described extensively – focuses on improving the whole experience of that product or service in terms of how it looks and feels). Take either the experience or the participatory stream away and there is no EBD.

There is an extensive literature relating to the first stream – participatory design (PD) – which we briefly summarise here as it plays such a prominent part in the case study. PD is commonly defined as:

> *an approach to the assessment, design and development of technological and organisational systems that places a premium on the active involvement of workplace practitioners (usually potential or current users of the system) in design and decision-making processes.*[38]

PD was first used in work on the design of computer systems in collaboration with Scandinavian trade unions in the 1960s and 1970s[39,40] and is characterised by the interaction between practical understanding and creation[41] with the aim of enabling design experts to gain the practical understanding they need for successful design. While there are a wide range of approaches to PD it typically involves users playing a central role in the design of new technologies or products – in particular, telling designers about their work environments and the tasks they are trying to accomplish, including what works for them and what does not when they use their current tools. Suchman puts it nicely when describing PD as a perspective with a concern for a 'more humane, creative and effective relationship between those involved in technology's design and its use'.[42]

Participatory and collaborative approaches to change are obviously no stranger to OD or service improvement, particularly in a healthcare setting,[43,44] but the notion of systems, product and service design for, with, and by the users[45] takes this involvement a step further, together with a completely new emphasis on user participation rather than the more usual staff participation found in OD.[46] Being action and improvement focused (what works and will work) means that explanation and reasoning within this highly participative setting take second place to active solution finding. Contemporary parallel initiatives in healthcare include the growing field of community-based participatory research (CBPR)[47] as we have already mentioned (*see* page 9). Generally, however, existing mechanisms for fully involving patients and carers in the design of healthcare services seem woefully inadequate (*see*, for example, Buchanan and colleagues[48] whose work we have already referenced briefly, and Wright and colleagues who make the point in their paper on participatory research in setting cancer research priorities[49] of the relatively limited level of patient involvement that currently exists); organisational, professional and data-related factors limiting the impact of patient survey data on quality improvement efforts have similarly been reported.[50] This is an issue we return to in more detail in Chapter 10.

Sitting at the other extreme is participatory co-design which, we need to stress from the outset, while offering scope for extensive patient and user participation, is still not 'patient-led' as such. The 'co' prefix in co-design in this instance suggests more of a partnership, with internal staff and users meeting and engaging in 'service dialogues'[4] with each other as they search for new and innovative ways to improve a product or service. At the same time it does not mean trying to make the users into design – or, for that matter, change – 'experts', but having them there precisely because they are the consumers not the experts, the 'lead users' rather than leaders,[51] with that precious and very special kind of first-hand knowledge and lay expertise we call experience. Hence co-design is an extension of the traditional 'influence continuum' that takes user involvement one step further on (*see* Figure 1.2, page 10) but stops short of control, or, in the case of our particular area of work, of a 'patient-led service'; a term full of good intentions but one that, in our view, betrays the naivety of much contemporary thinking around the idea of user involvement in healthcare, and has had the unfortunate effect of frightening many people off.

References

1 Berry LL, Wall EA, Carbone LP. Service clues and customer assessment of the service experience: lessons from marketing. *Academy of Management Perspectives.* 2006; **20**(2): 55.

2 Charmaz K, Mitchell RG. Grounded theory in ethnography. In: Atkinson P, Coffey A, Delamont S *et al.*, editors. *Handbook of Ethnography.* London: Sage; 2001.

3 Bergson H. *An Introduction to Metaphysics.* (Andison ML, trans., from 1903 original.) New York: Philosophical Library; 1961.

4 Forlizzi J, Battarbee K. Understanding experiences in interactive systems. Proceedings of the DIS04 Conference; 2004 August; Cambridge, MA.

5 Geertz C. *The Interpretation of Cultures.* New York: Basic Books; 1973.

6 Martin D, Rouncefield M, Sommerville I. Applying patterns of cooperative interaction to work (re)design: E-government and planning. In: Proceedings of the SIGCHI Conference on Human Factors; 2002.

7 Bate SP. Whatever happened to organisational anthropology? A review of the field of organisational ethnography and anthropological studies. *Human Relations.* 1997; **50**(9): 1147–75.

8 Lett J. Emic/etic distinctions. http://faculty.ircc.edu/faculty/jlett/Article%20on% 20Emics%20and%20Etics.htm (accessed 13 June 2006).

9 Van Maanen J. *Tales of the Field: On Writing Ethnography.* Chicago, IL: University of Chicago Press; 1988. p. 2.

10 Van Maanen J. Different strokes: qualitative research in the Administrative Science Quarterly from 1956 to 1996. In: Van Maanen J, editor. *Qualitative Studies of Organisations.* Thousand Oaks, CA: Sage; 1998. p. ix–xxxii.

11 Battarbee K. Defining co-experience. Proceedings of the 2003 DPPI'03 International Conference on Designing Pleasurable Products and Interfaces; 2003 June 23–26; Pittsburgh, PA, USA.

12 Forlizzi J, Ford S. The building blocks of experience: an early framework for interaction designers. Proceedings of the Conference on Designing Interactive Systems: Processes, Methods and Techniques; 2000 August; New York City, NY, USA.

13 Lauer Q. *Phenomenology: Its Genesis and Prospect.* New York: Harper Torchbooks; 1958.

14 Bourdieu P. Understanding. *Theory, Culture and Society.* 1996; **13**(2): 17–37.

15 Fulton Suri J. Empathetic design: informed and inspired by other people's experience. In: Koskinen I, Batterbee K, Mattelmaki T, editors. *Empathetic Design – User Experience in Product Design.* Helsinki: IT Press; 2003. p. 51–8.

16 Burch R. Phenomenology, lived experience: taking a measure of the topic. *Phenomenology and Pedagogy.* 2005; **8**: 130–60.

17 Kissell J. Phenomenonology. The science of experience. 6 July 2004. http://itotd.com/ index.alt?ArticleID=237 (accessed 2 August 2006).

18 Laurel B. Narrative construction as play. *Interactions.* 2004; **11**(5): 73–4.

19 Mäkelä A, Giller V, Tscheligi M *et al.* Joking, storytelling, artsharing, expressing affection: a field trial of how children and their social network communicate with digital

images in leisure time. Proceedings of the SIGCHI Conference on Human Factors in Computing Systems; 2000 April 1–6; The Hague, The Netherlands. p. 548–55.

20 Benford S, Bederson B, Akesson K *et al.* Designing storytelling technologies to encourage collaboration between young children. Proceedings of Human Factors in Computing Systems; 2000.

21 Stanton D, Bayon V, Neale H *et al.* Classroom collaboration in the design of tangible interfaces for storytelling. Proceedings of the SIGCHI Conference on Human Factors; 2001.

22 Ehn P, Kyng M. Cardboard computers: mock-it up or hands-on the future. In: Greenbaum J, Kyng M, editors. *Design at Work: Cooperative Design of Computer Systems.* Hillsdale, NJ: Lawrence Erlbaum; 1991.

23 Dewey J. *Art as Experience.* London: The Berkeley Publishing Group; 1934.

24 Boland RJ, Collopy F. Managing as designing: bringing the art of design to the practice of management. (DVD.) Information Design Studio, Case Western University, Weatherhead School of Management; 2004. *See* also Sydney Pollack's recent film documentary *Sketches of Frank Gehry*, DVD, Sony Pictures, released 22 August 2006.

25 Monk A, Hassenzahl M, Blythe M *et al.* Funology: designing enjoyment. Proceedings of CHI2002; 2002 April 20–25; Minneapolis, MN: ACM 1–58113–454–1/02/0004.

26 Cooperrider DL, Whitney D. A positive revolution in change: Appreciative Inquiry. In: Cooperrider DL, Sorenson PF, Whitney D *et al.*, editors. *Appreciative Inquiry.* Champaign, IL: Stipes; 2000. p. 3–28.

27 Cameron KS, Dutton JE, Quinn RE, editors. *Positive Organisational Scholarship: Foundations of a New Discipline.* San Francisco, CA: Berrett-Koehler; 2003.

28 Draper SW. Analysing fun as a candidate software requirement. *Personal Technology.* 1999; **3**(1): 1–6.

29 Hobbs D, May T, editors. *Interpreting the Field. Accounts of Ethnography.* Oxford: Clarenden Press; 1993.

30 Bate SP. Changing the culture of a hospital: from hierarchy to networked community. *Public Administration.* 2000; **78**(3): 485–512.

31 Bate SP, Khan R, Pye A. Towards a culturally sensitive approach to organisation structuring: where organisation design meets organisation development. *Organisation Science.* 2000; **11**(2): 197–211.

32 Bate SP, Robert G. Towards more user-centric organisational development: lessons from a case study of experience-based design. *Journal of Applied Behavioral Science.* 2007; **43**(1): 41–66.

33 Bloor M. The ethnography of health and medicine. In: Atkinson P, Coffey A, Delamont S *et al.*, editors. *Handbook of Ethnography.* London: Sage; 2001. p. 177–87.

34 Goffman E. *Asylums: Essays on the Social Situation of Mental Patients and Other Inmates.* New York: Doubleday Anchor; 1961.

35 Strauss AL, Fagerhaugh S, Suczek B *et al. Social Organization of Medical Work.* Chicago: University of Chicago; 1985.

36 Roth J. *Timetables: Structuring the Passage of Time in Hospital Treatment and Other Careers.* New York: Bobbs Merrill; 1963.

37 Becker HS, Geer B, Hughes EC *et al. Boys in White: Student Culture in Medical School.* Chicago: University of Chicago Press; 1961.

38 Computer Professionals for Social Responsibility. Participatory design. www.cpsr.org/issues/pd/index_html/view?searchterm=participatory%20design (accessed 21 July 2006).

39 Floyd C, Mehl W-M, Reisin F-M *et al.* Out of Scandinavia: alternative approaches to software design and system development. *Human-Computer Interaction.* 1989; **4**(4): 253–350.

40 Clement A, Besselaar PVd. A retrospective look at PD projects. *Communications of the ACM.* 1993; **36**(4): 29–39.

41 Ehn P. Scandinavian design: on participation and skill. In: Schuler D, Namioka A, editors. *Participatory Design: Principles and Practices*. Hillsdale, NJ: Lawrence Erlbaum Associates; 1993. p. 41–77.

42 Suchman L. Foreword. In: Schuler D, Namioka A, editors. *Participatory Design: Principles and Practices*. Hillsdale, NJ: Lawrence Erlbaum Associates; 1993.

43 Bragg JE, Andrews IR. Participative decision-making: an experimental study in a hospital. *Journal of Applied Behavioral Science*. 1973; **9**(6): 727–35.

44 Boss W. *Organization Development in Health Care*. Reading, MA: Addison-Wesley; 1989.

45 Briefs U, Ciborra C, Schneider L, editors. *Systems Design For, With and By the Users*. Amsterdam: North-Holland; 1983.

46 Bartunek JM, Greenberg DN, Davidson B. Consistent and inconsistent impacts of a teacher-led empowerment initiative in a federation of schools. *Journal of Applied Behavioral Science*. 1999; **35**(4): 457–78.

47 Minkler M, Wallerstein N, editors. *Community-Based Participatory Research for Health*. New York, NY: Jossey-Bass; 2003.

48 Buchanan D, Abbott S, Bentley J *et al*. Let's be PALS: user-driven organisational change in healthcare. *British Journal of Management*. 2005; **16**(4): 315–28.

49 Wright D, Corner J, Hopkinson J *et al*. Listening to the views of people affected by cancer about cancer research: an example of participatory research in setting the cancer research agenda. *Health Expectations*. 2006; **9**: 3–12.

50 Davies E, Cleary PD. Hearing the patient's voice? Factors affecting the use of patient survey data in quality improvement. *Quality and Safety in Health Care*. 2005; **14**: 428–32.

51 Von Hippel E. *Democratising Innovation*. Cambridge, MA: The MIT Press; 2005.

Chapter 6

Using stories and storytelling to reveal the users'-eye view of the landscape

We grasp our lives in a narrative ... Making sense of one's life as a story is not an optional extra. Our lives exist also in this space of questions, which only a coherent narrative can answer. (Charles Taylor)

Language alone brings what is, as something that is, into the open for the first time. (Martin Heidegger)

There is no lived experience without language and no language without lived experience. (Robert Burch)

We understand the world largely through narrative construction. (Michael Mateas and Phoebe Sengers)

Narrative and stories as the wings of experience

Narrative and stories, oral or written, are far and away the most powerful and natural way of accessing human experience, and it is therefore no surprise to find them in rapidly growing professional use in contemporary medicine and medical research.[1] Once again, we believe that ethnography can take much of the credit for this.[2,3] Cortazzi writes:

> *There is increasing recognition of the importance and usefulness of narrative analysis as an element of doing ethnography. This is hardly surprising. Narrative is now seen as one of the fundamental ways in which humans organise their understanding of the world. Most social science and human disciplines have recently turned to narrative analysis for the human involvement in reporting an evaluating experience. Narrating is, after all, a major means of making sense of past experience and sharing it with others.*[2]

As already suggested, what makes the narrative–experience link so strategically important in experience design is that it is not possible to access experiences directly, and therefore one is obliged to do this indirectly by focusing on the words people use to organise, describe, make sense and communicate them. Narrative is the means whereby people share *the meaning of experience*. Thus Polkinghorne (cited by Cortazzi[2]) defines narrative as 'the primary scheme by means of which human existence is rendered meaningful'. Similarly Bruner defines narrative as the 'organising principle' by which people 'organise their experience in, knowledge about, and transactions with the social world'.[2] Branigan's view is also very similar: he defines narrative as 'a perceptual activity that organises data into a special pattern which represents and explains experience'.[2] White[2] claims that narratives translate knowing into telling, hence telling gets us back to sense-making, sense-making back to knowing, and knowing back to experiencing.

Unfortunately, some of the impact of the above quotations is lost in their somewhat obtuse language, and therefore a more effective way of thinking about the narrative–experience link would be to stop and reflect on some of your favourite books or poems, fact or fiction. It is then that you realise that all the rich and memorable experiences they contain are no more than black squiggles on a page (or, orally, noises from the mouth). That is the beauty and functionality of words – they capture reality in flight, and equally they hold it until you are ready to access it. 'Words', as Crescimanno put it so wonderfully, 'are the wings of meaning'.[4]

Even better, read some of the gripping, gut-wrenching, sensual, sometimes violent and sickening true-life stories in books like Ellis and Bochner's *Composing Ethnography*[5] to feel the full weight and power of narrative as a medium for communicating experience: Lisa Tillman-Healy's story of her lifelong and never-ending battle with bulimia, written with the aim of producing a 'sensual text' that would take you into the experience of how bulimia *feels*;[6] Carol Rambo Ronai's account of her life with a mentally retarded mother whom she loved as one would any other mother but who sexually abused her or delivered her to her father for him to do the same ('What is it like to live through an experience that potentially places you in a muddle of uncertainty, doubt, contradiction, and ambivalence?');[7] Aliza Kolker's story of her personal, ongoing war against breast cancer ('My body has been violated and mutilated, and the violations are escalating. First I lost my hair, then my eyebrows and body hair, then my breast. Now I have two plastic pipes about eight inches long hanging out of my chest. I am aware this is just the beginning of the illness odyssey. It's amazing what a human being can tolerate');[8] Caroline Ellis' story of nursing her incontinent mother in hospital;[9] and Karen's Fox's stories of child sexual abuse, including her own, in which she notes with admirable understatement that child abuse researchers are still not studying the lived experiences of the victims, or for that matter the perpetrators, but remain closeted away in the safe, emotionally disinfected zone of rational science.[10] As Van Maanen comments: 'ethnographies are portraits of diversity in an increasingly homogenous world',[11] portraits that are not only deeply moving but also insightful and informative from the point of view of service improvement and change. Through them we can begin to appreciate why the subject of anthropology was invented in the first place as an 'antidote' to science (or, if you prefer, the more formal 'romantic rebellion against the enlightenment'), its early protagonists driven by the conviction that there were other, equally valid, ways of 'knowing' the world than offered by the lens of science. Equally today, these stories are a reminder that there are other ways of addressing service development and change that should not have to continue to rely solely on the 'science of improvement'.

Stories of medicine and illness

It is no coincidence that most of the examples in Ellis and Bochner's book are stories of medicine and illness. This is reflected in the wider literature on narrative and storytelling, which includes masterpieces such as Sandra Butler and Barbara Rosenblum's *Cancer in Two Voices*[12] and Marianne Paget's book *A Complex Sorrow*[13] (all three authors were to die of cancer before they could complete their work) and many more. For a comprehensive review of the ethnographic literature on narratives of illness and health, readers should consult Kolker.[8] For a fuller exploration of the ethnography of subjectivity and experience, again including healthcare examples like issues of choice in abortion, readers might also wish to see Ellis and Flaherty,[14] Denzin,[15] and Denzin and Lincoln.[16]

Healthcare is thus blessed with some of the best ethnographic narratives ever written. Of course, these are mostly stories written by professional writers (proper name 'autoethnography'); we will need to ask later whether non-professional writers are at a disadvantage, or whether anyone can talk or write naturally and lucidly about their own experiences – or be able to acquire the skill to do so. For the moment all we are doing is trying to highlight the power of narrative in conveying all aspects of the life experience – feelings and emotions, thoughts and perceptions, behaviour and conduct.

This is particularly true of the more dramatic, epiphanic moments in life[2] – crises, highs and lows, and matters of love, relationships, career and health. A good illustration is Deborah Wearing's recent moving account of how, as the result of a brain virus, her musician husband became trapped, memoryless, in the limbo of the constant present ('life outside time'), and yet how they were able to partly conquer the illness with a bond of love which, as she puts it, ran deeper than conscious thought.[17] Another is Ben Watt's remarkable book about his own illness (necrotic bowel and complications) and two and a half month hospitalisation, much of this time spent in intensive care (or intensive therapy unit, ITU) where on a number of occasions he came very close to death.[18] In the light of what has just been said about the skill of storytelling, it is reassuring to find that Watt is a singer (in fact lead singer of the 1980s pop band Everything But the Girl) not a professional writer; his and Wearing's book offering proof that one does not have to be an anthropologist to produce a compelling, moving and intense narrative of one's own experiences.

One could have selected any number of illustrative extracts from Watt's book, but the one that follows is a good example of what Geertz called the 'being-there' quality of a narrative account, because of its ability to transport the reader into the ward or department where the action took place, even into the body and mind of the patient himself or those around him, and to convey the whole experience fresh and in the raw. More than this, the narrative is dripping with information about how services might be redesigned and improved for others in Ben's position in the future. It all leaves one wondering how experience-rich narratives like this could possibly have been ignored in traditional service redesign for so long:

> *Like a lone diver among sharks, I would watch the cool-eyed doctors and anaesthetists glide round my bed. The doctors on ITU were strange, humourless, intent. They struck me as total scientists – more so than any doctors I came across. Most of the patients they were treating were living on the slope of death. Patient survival was rooted in the minute analysis of charts and the balancing of chemicals, not so much in the warmth of human contact, and so the doctors glided from flickering monitor to flickering monitor amid the sonars of bleeps and alarms, gauging, estimating, quiet, serious. I never struck up a conversation with one of them, just gleaned a few facts and watched them mutter among themselves . . .*
>
> *Henry, an old man opposite me, slept all the time, unhappy on his respirator, beyond the tree line of consciousness for hours on end. When he woke he couldn't speak, and would toss his head around on the pillow. One nurse told me that he'd lost the will to live and often wouldn't even try to breathe, needing reprimands and chest massages. He'd let the female nurses wash him but he'd never let them shave him . . .*

I felt like a child on a bunk-bed. I was wearing a cotton theatre robe, stiff and starched, tied in bows down the back. Everybody I saw who wore one standing up felt their arse was on show and that everyone was looking. I used to watch wide-eyed out-patients and newcomers pulling the material together behind them, covering up, grasping at their dignity. Theatre gowns are a cruel design, playing on the quiet humiliation brought on by unfamiliar hospital life. They level everyone. Hospital turns life upside down. It seems fitting that the uniform should be a gown worn back to front . . .

The steel trolley-frame was cold against the back of my thighs. All my lines had been removed. I felt relaxed. The black cup came. I breathed in the oxygen. The veins in my arms were dry river-beds and I had no lines, so the needle for the anaesthetic had to be twice jammed in deep before the blood table was found. It felt like a big needle. In my mind's eye I saw oilrigs, derricks out at sea, the huge spinning drills spitting oil, churning, billowing waves, grey and green, the colours of nausea . . . The anaesthetist mumbled behind his mask. I closed my eyes. 'One, two . . .' Hummingbirds, hummingbirds . . . 'three, four, fi' . . . Gone.

I am lying on my side. Why my side? Who rolled me over? The cotton blanket is warm. The trolley is hard. I am frightened to move lest I disturb the surgeon's work. Or cause pain. Fresh, crisp, newly made pain. The light is bright and even and white all over the room. It is like opening a fridge door. A nurse sits at a table. Other trolleys. Other sleeping patients on their sides. Not many. I can see two. I am thirsty. I think I want to shit. I move a little. A little test. My chest hurts. I stop moving. I close my eyes and press my nose into the cotton blanket. Rest and sleep. A good place. Save me.

The staff nurse asks me to sit up. I say I can't. She says, 'Try.' I say I haven't been able to sit up on my own for three weeks. She says I have to. 'This isn't ITU any more. This is the road to recovery.' Another nurse comes over. They slip their arms under my armpits and each puts one knee on the bed. 'Sit forward.' I try. They heave me forward. I cry out. They hold me there. I am limp, like a puppy in its mother's mouth, but there is dreadful, dreadful pain. So bad, I have no breath. I can't draw in breath to speak. I open and close my mouth like a fish. I want to say, 'Stop.'

This narrative, and others like it, contain so much of the raw material for design – still 'raw', however, since the narrative materials don't just design themselves into better care processes. What this needs is the design process itself, which takes something (in this case an experience) that happened in the past and fashions it into something for the future. Words without a design process are just words, talk but not design.

Analysing narrative and stories: a primer

Later, we shall be proposing various ways for systematically analysing – deconstructing – narrative like this, and then reconstructing it through a design process, first into a model or prototype, and then into the real thing. Before leaving Ben, however, it might be worth flagging up one or two parts from his story that narrative-design specialists would almost certainly be focusing on in their improvement efforts. These include narrative references that have implications for the design of the social system (roles, interactions and behaviour), the physical and technical environment, and the aesthetics of the patient's experience.

- *'I never struck up a conversation with one of them, just gleaned a few facts and watched them mutter among themselves.'* (social)

Comment: Ben obviously feels isolated from the doctors around him, and generally excluded from ITU ward life. He feels part of a dehumanising treatment regime, mediated by high technology, which puts him on the 'receiving end' of treatment. He feels exposed and unsafe ('a lone diver among sharks'). His experience flies in the face of recent microsystems literature which has demonstrated that patients' experience significantly improves when they are treated as *members* or citizens of the clinical microsystem, not merely the passive recipients of care.[19,20] In this case, Ben implies that his experience might have been transformed if he had been treated less like a marginal native and more like a member of the ITU community.

- *'I used to watch wide-eyed out-patients and newcomers pulling the material together behind them, covering up, grasping at their dignity. Theatre gowns are a cruel design, playing on the quiet humiliation brought on by unfamiliar hospital life.'* (physical artefact)

Comment: The hospital gown: that old chestnut that everybody talks about but still remains standard issue in healthcare. Even as we write there is someone somewhere feeling infantilised, embarrassed and humiliated by it. As Ben says, it is a 'cruel design'. Consider how much better the patient experience would be if someone could come up with a gown that preserves people's modesty and self-esteem, or even looks quite trendy and fashionable, but still did the job (P + E + A). The question for co-design is: is this what a patient would have come up with if he or she had been invited to design the gown? Clearly not. Here is a classic case of something that scores quite highly on functionality (P, easy to remove in the operating theatre, etc.) but zero in term of interactivity (have you tried tying the bows at the back?) and aesthetics of experience (A).

- *'The steel trolley-frame was cold against the back of my thighs'.* . . . [and later in recovery] *'The trolley is hard.'* (physical object)

Comment: So how might the trolley be redesigned to make it warmer and more comfortable? Considerations would include other features like the bars at the sides, designed to stop you falling out, but leaving you feeling like a caged animal or back in the play-pen. Typically designers seeking to improve the 'trolley experience' would think and talk through various alternatives and then pilot and field-test these by constructing various low- and high-fidelity prototypes (*see* later). The value patients and staff would bring to this process does not even need stating, but clearly they were not present when the trolley was first designed.

- *'The light is bright and even and white all over the room. It is like opening a fridge door.'* (environment/aesthetics)

Comment: How might the aesthetics be improved so that the physical environment one is waking up to feels less stark and 'fridge-like'? It must be possible to design easier and more pleasant ways of coming round, including not only better environmental aesthetics but more human contact, so that Ben feels less isolated and alone.

- *'The staff nurse asks me to sit up. I say I can't. She says, 'Try.' I say I haven't been able to sit up on my own for three weeks. She says I have to. 'This isn't ITU any more. This is the road to recovery.'* (interactions)

Comment: From a design point of view there are myriad issues here around attitudes (might the nurses have adopted a different, less brusque, attitude towards him?), behaviour (were there other ways in which they might have done this, or is it really a case of having to be cruel to be kind?), and script (could they have said different things that would have made Ben feel less apprehensive about sitting up, and more convinced that this really was the road to recovery?). Focusing on interactions like this does not necessarily imply that it can or should be changed. This is an example of 'bracketing' an habitual, taken-for-granted mindset and set of practices and merely asking: are there things that might be changed here that would make the patient experience of the first steps towards mobility and recovery less painful and unpleasant?

Part of the challenge in listening to and deciphering stories like Ben's is being aware of what is *absent* from a patient's account of his or her experience – what Sherlock Holmes famously described as 'the dog that didn't bark in the night'. One absentee in Ben's case, and not unusually, is humour. Ben's story reminds us that hospitals, for patients at least, can be pretty humourless places, and hardly the place to go for a revival of the spirits. Of course illness is a serious business, but experience designers would still argue that things that make people laugh are not disrespectful, but part of the healing process. The importance of humour in experience and experience design has recently been highlighted by Bob Mankoff, the cartoon editor of the *New Yorker*, speaking about his three-year research project with academics in the psychology department of the University of Michigan, in the experience design newsletter, *Gel*. Mankoff points out that humour shares its cognitive apparatus with 99% of other brain processes, and that it is the additional 1% that makes things look completely different.[21] By the same token, that 1% in Ben's story might have made his experience of the hospital completely different.

For this reason, humour, pleasure and fun must be included along with the other emotional elements as a legitimate and valuable part of the design process and experience. This does not have to mean Sister walking around wearing a red nose (an interesting thought!) or the surgeon cracking tasteless jokes about taking off the wrong leg, merely designing (stress 'designing') ways of using humour and fun in positive ways to relax, entertain, distract, and de-stress patients, and to help begin to instil feelings of hope and optimism.

No matter how powerful and rich in 'design insight' stories like Ben Watt's are, they are still often viewed with deep suspicion by scientists and clinicians alike. After all, accounts like these are just not 'scientific' (and therefore not valid)!

> *I suspect stories, in particular, haven't been discussed much because they aren't . . . well stories aren't very respectable. Stories are subjective. Stories are ambiguous. Stories are particular. They are at odds with the scientific drive towards objective, generalisable, respectable findings.*[22]

We believe this situation is rapidly changing. For example, Hurwitz and colleagues' recent book collection contains many stories actually written by clinicians.[1] Nevertheless, we do subscribe to Neumann's view that 'academic conventions have constrained rather than enabled the representation of subjective experience',[23] including the use of narrative and storytelling.

The point of stories

Actually, this is the very point of stories, which are not gathered because they are assumed to be objective, accurate or verifiable but because they are uniquely human and subjective, describing not a fact or a reality but a recalled experience or set of experiences. Located firmly within this subjective, socially constructed world, EBD involves interacting and working – literally co-designing – with these subjectivities, words being the basic currency of that interaction and the raw material of interpretation. Through personal stories and anecdote, users reveal what they like about a service (or healthcare in general), what they hate about it, what matters to them, works well for them, and what sorts of things cause real anxieties or problems, as well as comfort and reassurance. Such stories and anecdotes might be unique, one-off events, but they will also connect branch and root to deeper, wider and more permanent meanings, assumptions, values, expectations, cognitions and emotions, which are the actual target of EBD, not so much experiences.

Stories are the structure, sense and significance given to the experience *by those whose experience it is*, free of any external structure or meaning imposed by others. People do of course alter, embellish, exaggerate, or simply make things up – all stories being to some extent confabulations or fictionalisations of reality (for as Burch notes '. . . in our explicit reflection we are as apt to tell ourselves "tales" in order, for example, to salvage our pride or sanity'[24]) – but this is not as big a problem as one might think, since whatever they say will provide useful and valid information as to how they might wish or have wished to experience the service on another occasion. Again, it is 'truth-value' for the user not truth *per se* that one is after. At the same time, stories are the means whereby we store a memory, and therefore when we listen to a story we are in fact tapping into that memory, and being given the privilege of sharing the action replay.

The term 'narrative' covers a wide range of types of talk and text, and one of the fundamental distinctions is whether they are something intended to be listened to (of the church or Alcoholics Anonymous confessional, conference presentation or stage performance variety), or part of an ongoing discursive interaction and joint production between two or more people. Both are valuable in ethnography and design, and both involve somewhat different methods and processes. The first is a useful reminder that there does not need to be intense interaction every time for a narrative to be useful or usable. Just telling or listening to someone else's story can help one understand his or her, or even one's own, experience, and to learn what needs to be done differently in the future. In this case the method is one of *narrative analysis* for service design, whereas the second, being more of an interactive co-production between teller and listener, is much closer to *conversational analysis*[25] and co-design. At this group conversational level, storytelling can be a highly effective way of stimulating the design process, since when told publicly the stories invariably evoke strong reactions, as people nod, laugh or cry, and ultimately begin to open up and tell their own stories. As our later case study shows, frequently as a result of this, the design process acquires its own energy, and begins to run itself with minimal intervention from the facilitators (in OD the term is 'autocatalytic' or self-fuelling).

The design process can benefit from stories in other ways. For example, the tone and atmosphere created by stories, by their very nature, is attractively equal and democratic. People are not setting themselves up as experts or judges, merely telling what happened to them in a language that anyone can understand, hence the additional benefit of having a largely jargon and expert-free process. As Erickson puts it:

> *Stories are a sort of equaliser. It doesn't require much expertise or training to listen to and tell stories. Team members from any background can be made part of the process of telling and collecting stories. And once stories have been gathered, team members can discuss the stories, argue about their interpretation, and generate hypotheses about what are users' problems, needs and practices. This process sensitises everyone to usage domain, helps people identify questions and issues to probe for when they talk with users, and best of all provides concrete examples which can prove invaluable when team discussions threaten to veer into debates about vaguely defined abstractions.*[26]

As our fieldwork with EBD has shown, stories, spoken or written, come in all shapes and sizes: 'war stories',[27] vignettes, even romances, which take in the full sweep from the tragic to the comedic (yes, even some cancer stories can be funny). Some are short, punchy and down to earth (Geertz has a fancy but nice term for them: he calls these 'ethnographic miniatures'[28]), while others – the legends for example – are often long and lofty, heroic and ultimately uplifting ('winning my battle against cancer'). Then there are epic sagas (which are positively oozing with cultural insight – *see* below), evocative narratives about brave and courageous exploits performed in the face of adversity: 'They are the ideological parables that express, enhance, and codify beliefs'.[29] Van Maanen also prepares us for different kinds of stories:[30] the 'realist tale' (sticks to the facts; this as far as I can best remember is what happened and happened in this order); the 'confessional tale' (this is what happened warts and all, and this is how I felt about all of it); and the 'impressionist tale', a sort of caricature or impression of what happened, a dab here, a dab there. (Again we have been surprised how many patients will miss out or skate over large parts of their stories, not because of some kind of lapse or repression of memory but because they don't consider them to be of sufficient significance or importance to their overall experience. That is the thing about stories; it is the storyteller who decides what is significant and important, nobody else.) Some stories are about what worked well (appreciative stories) while others describe things that were problematic or just went badly wrong. All of these stories, no matter what particular category or type, contain huge amounts of information, wisdom and intelligence about experiences that are waiting to be tapped as a rich source for future service development and design. For example, stories will typically help us to identify some of the following:

- problem and issue definitions
- opportunities and quick-wins
- key 'touch points', the 'experience hot spots' (good and bad) towards which interventions will need to be directed
- lists and rich descriptions of user needs and perceptions
- a list of design patterns or principles ('must do's or 'must be's for the future process – *see* Chapter 7)
- prototypes for the new process.

Summary

Stories and storytelling are the basis of experience design. They are a rich source of learning about people's experiences, and will contain most of the things that will be required to gain a deep appreciative understanding of the strengths and weaknesses of a present service and what is needed for the future (for the connection between learning, narrative and EBD *see* Alger[31]). Making the case for 'narratively competent medicine' (of which we would argue EBD is an important part) Rita Charon sums up a lot of what we have been trying to say in this chapter about the transformative potential of narrative and storytelling, and its ability to 'fix things that do not yet work':

> *Sickness unfolds in stories. Whether in a patient's chief complaint, a family member's saga of surgery, an intern's presentation at attending rounds, or a death note in a chart, the events of illness unfurl and accrue meaning by being told. Equipping health professionals with the wherewithal to recognise, absorb and be moved by the stories patients tell – might go a long way toward fixing what doesn't yet work in medicine.*
>
> *Narratively competent medicine – or narrative medicine for short – recognises patients' needs to tell of their illness in order to comprehend it . . . Narrative skills help to bring us near patients in professional engagement instead of detached concern.*[32]

We would go further to reiterate that there is no substitute for storytelling as far as a number of things are concerned: the natural and easy access it gives we the designers and the participants themselves to their experiences; the way it can help equalise the co-design process, even where there is considerable hierarchical distance (as often in EBD) between those involved, and provide it with its own internal source of energy; and finally, a point still to be covered, how the story once heard can compel us to *have* to take action – to make change a personal imperative, an inner, self-imposed, as opposed to outer, requirement. The story does not allow us to opt out or adopt the position of 'detached concern' referred to by Charon; we have to engage whether we like it or not; we are entrapped by the story.

As ever, these various 'qualities' of the story cannot be dealt with adequately at the abstract level but have to be experienced directly for themselves. We have already had a taste of this with Ben's story but will end with another true story, related to us by Barbara Monroe, Chief Executive of St Christopher's Hospice in South London, which communicates the painful and desperately sad experience of a family faced with a terminally ill member:

> *. . . a young woman with breast cancer, multiple secondaries, and her husband and two children. She says, 'I don't want to die in hospital'. He says, 'I don't think she should have any more chemotherapy'. She is trying every experimental treatment she can at the local hospital because she wants to carry on living. She's got kids. He says, 'She won't face it, we need a nanny now, because she's going blind', because she's got secondaries just behind her eyes. She says, 'Can I trust him with the children?' She says, 'I need to stay alive for as long as possible'. One day when I was visiting them, they completely knocked me over because she looked at me and she said, 'Have you got any suggestions for*

improving our sex life?' This is a woman who's had a double mastectomy, who's skeletal, who's got a problem with uncontrolled vomiting. I wasn't even thinking about their sex life or that they were thinking about their sex life, but for them this was a really important way of staying connected as a couple.

They had two children: 'Why can't the nurses make her better?' Despite the fact that she wanted to die at home, in fact, her brain secondaries in the last two or three days of her life meant that in the end her husband decided that he couldn't continue to look after her at home. The children were with her and in her room at the hospice when she died, and the room was a four-bedded bay. I shall never forget being with these two children, aged four and six, and the four-year-old said, 'She's resting'. The six-year-old said very loudly, 'No, she's not, she's snuffed it'. And there are three other dying people just beyond the curtains and I thought, 'Oh, how do you make this okay?' In fact, the other three people, when I went to talk to them, all said how glad they were that these children were able to be with their mum at such an important time.

Next day they're visiting, they're going to collect the death certificate, they're going to pick up mum's belongings, and they visit mum's body: 'Is she completely dead?' 'Will she still be dead when I'm 10, when I'm 15?' 'Why is daddy crying?' 'Why is mummy cold?' We'd just got mummy out of our fridge and the kids were touching her and she was a bit slicky, the way bodies are when they come out of the fridge. And then they look at their dad and they say, 'Will you keep one side of the bed for mummy's ghost?' This man who's grieving who has just had his wife die also has to try and manage his children and their very practical questions. It was just before Christmas. Kids know that daddy won't get the Christmas presents right. 'Can we come to the funeral?' 'What happens when your heart stops?' 'When will daddy die?' 'Who's more important, God or Jesus?' 'What are spirits?' 'Who goes to Hell?' As it happens, these kids had a cat that was called Black Cat, and by a horrible coincidence Black Cat had cancer. And just to remind us that there isn't some recipe book of skills, and I've been in the business for quite a long time, but these kids looked at me and said, 'They're going to kill Black Cat. Nobody put mummy to sleep. Why don't they put people to sleep if they put animals to sleep?' I didn't know the answer to that so I said, 'I don't know'.

Stories like this remind us that there is so much more to stories and storytelling than design, that they also hold the key to the humanisation of health services (which necessarily involves a design process anyway). One source has put it this way: 'In a field of practice criticised for the many ways it can dehumanise and detach, storytelling in health care helps to personalise and connect'.[33] John Steinbeck, the writer, put it even better:

We are lonesome animals. We spend all our life trying to be less lonesome. One of our ancient methods is to tell a story begging the listener to say – and to feel – 'Yes, that is the way it is, or at least the way I feel it.' You're not as alone as you thought.[34]

References

1 Hurwitz B, Greenhalgh T, Skultans V, editors. *Narrative Research in Health and Illness.* London: BMJ Publications; 2004.

2 Cortazzi M. Narrative analysis in ethnography. In: Atkinson P, Coffey A, Delamont S *et al.*, editors. *Handbook of Ethnography*. London: Sage; 2001. p. 384.

3 Hansen H. The ethnonarrative approach. *Human Relations*. 2006; **59**(8): 1049–75.

4 Crescimanno R. *Culture, Consciousness and Beyond*. Washington: University Press of America; 1982.

5 Ellis C, Bochner AP, editors. *Composing Ethnography: Alternative Forms of Qualitative Writing*. London: AltaMira Press; 1996.

6 Tillman-Healy L. A secret life in a culture of thinness: reflections on body, food and bulimia. In: Ellis C, Bochner AP, editors. *Composing Ethnography: Alternative Forms of Qualitative Writing*. London: AltaMira Press; 1996.

7 Ronai CR. On loving and hating my mentally retarded mother. *Mental Retardation*. 1997; **35** (6): 111.

8 Kolker A. Thrown overboard. In: Ellis C, Bochner AP, editors. *Composing Ethnography: Alternative Forms of Qualitative Writing*. London: AltaMira Press; 1996. p. 132–59.

9 Ellis C. *Final Negotiations: A Story of Love, Loss, and Chronic Illness*. Philadelphia: Temple University Press; 1995.

10 Fox KV. Silent voices, a subversive reading of child sexual abuse. In: Ellis C, Bochner AP, editors. *Composing Ethnography: Alternative Forms of Qualitative Writing*. London: AltaMira Press; 1996.

11 Van Maanen J. Different strokes: qualitative research in the Administrative Science Quarterly from 1956 to 1996. In: Van Maanen J, editor. *Qualitative Studies of Organisations*. Thousand Oaks, CA; Sage; 1998. p. xiii–iv.

12 Butler S, Rosenblum B. *Cancer in Two Voices*. San Francisco, CA: Spinsters Ink Books; 1991.

13 Paget M. *A Complex Sorrow: Reflections on Cancer and an Abbreviated Life*. Philadelphia: Temple University Press; 1993.

14 Ellis C, Flaherty M, editors. *Investigating Subjectivity: Research on Lived Experience*. Newbury Park, CA; Sage; 1992.

15 Denzin NK. Representing lived experience in ethnographic texts. In: Denzin NK, editor. *Studies in Symbolic Interactionism*, volume 12. Greenwich, CT: Jai Press; 1991. p. 59–70.

16 Denzin NK and Lincoln YS, editors. *Handbook of Qualitative Research*. Thousand Oaks, CA; Sage; 1994.

17 Wearing D. *Forever Today. A Memoir of Love and Amnesia*. London: Doubleday; 2005.

18 Watt B. *Patient: The True Story of a Rare Illness*. New York: Viking Press; 1998.

19 Mohr JJ, Batalden PB. Improving safety on the front lines: the role of clinical microsystems. *Quality and Safety in Health Care*. 2002; **11**: 45–50.

20 Nelson EC, Batalden PB, Huber TP *et al.* Microsystems in health care: Part 1. Learning from high-performing front-line clinical units. *Joint Commission Journal on Quality Improvement*. 2002; **29**(8): 472–93.

21 Good Experience. 8 April 2005. *See*: www.goodexperience.com (accessed 3 August 2006).

22 Erickson T. Notes on design practice: stories and prototypes as catalysts for communication. In: Carroll J, editor. *Scenario-Based Design: Envisioning Work and Technology in System Development*. New York; Wiley; 1995. p. 37–58.

23 Neumann M. Collecting ourselves at the end of the century. In: Ellis C, Bochner AP, editors. *Composing Ethnography: Alternative Forms of Qualitative Writing*. London: AltaMira Press; 1996. p. 193.

24 Burch R. Phenomenology, lived experience: taking a measure of the topic. *Phenomenology and Pedagogy*. 2005; **8**: 130–60.

25 Psathas G. *Conversation Analysis: The Study of Talk-In Interaction*. Thousand Oaks, CA: Sage; 1995.

26 Erickson T. Design as storytelling. *Interactions*. 1996; **3**(4): 30–5.

27 Orr J. *Talking About Machines: An Ethnography of a Modern Job*. Ithaca, NY: Cornell University Press; 1996.

28 Geertz C. *The Interpretation of Cultures*. New York: Basic Books; 1973.

29 Meyer AD. How ideologies supplant formal structures and shape responses to environments. *Journal of Management Studies*. 1982; **19**(1): 45–61.

30 Van Maanen J. *Tales of the Field: On Writing Ethnography*. Chicago: University of Chicago Press; 1988.

31 Alger B. *The Experience Designer: Learning, Networks and the Cybersphere*. Tucson, AZ: Fenestra Books; 2002.

32 Charon R. Fostering empathy. Narrative medicine offers new opportunities for practicing human medical care. *In Vivo*. 2003; **2**(12). www.cumc.columbia.edu/news/in-vivo/Vol2_Iss12_jul28_03/pov.html (accessed 7 December 2006).

33 Prescribing storytelling for health. Ivy Sea's Enlightened-Leadership Series. www.ivysea.com/pages/ca0701_2.html (accessed 3 August 2006).

34 Steinbeck J. In awe of words. *The Exonian*. 1954: **CCXXLV**. No. 14.

Chapter 7

Patterns-based design: the concept of 'design principles'

In studies of chess players asked to think aloud as they played, researchers discovered that expert players have a rich set of situation-dependent rules that guide their thinking. In the opening of the game, while novice players simply reacted to the moves of their opponent, expert players articulated a clear goal of wanting to gain superior positions on the board, and, therefore, moved in accordance with general plans such as 'try to maintain control of the central four squares on the board'. (Herbert Simon)

Patterns-based design belongs to the design field generally but in our view fits well with an EBD approach to healthcare improvement. The aim of this chapter is to say more about what patterns-based design is, how it relates to narratives and stories, the concepts and practices associated with it, and to prepare the reader for its application in the case study in Chapter 9.

The concept of design patterns or rules originates from two sources: the first, research into patterns in software engineering,[1] and the second, the work of architects and architectural design researchers like Christopher Alexander[2,3] and Lidwell and colleagues.[4] Organisational theorists have also just begun to explore and test 'design rules' as a means of reconnecting organisational science to organisational practice.[5] Plsek and colleagues[6] describe their experience in pilot tests of four different methods for extracting design rules from existing programmes of organisational change in the healthcare sector.

We should say here that we are happier with the concept of design patterns and principles than we are with design rules. 'Design rules' in an organisational as opposed to physical context seem too rigid and deterministic. What we are talking about here are only guides (guiding principles), not hard and fast rules, which say that 'if you try this, chances are it will work', not it will definitely work, or work every time. Alexander presents a pattern as *'a solution to a problem in context'*, which takes account of the relevant social and physical aspects of the setting. Through personal stories, recounted in our case by patients, staff and users (similar to the examples in the previous chapter), one seeks to discover the design patterns – the rules of thumb – upon which the present service is based, and which shape the everyday delivery of the service. These are the preferred solutions or 'recipes' which have evolved over time, and which are largely internalised and unconscious. Design patterns are important because they are, as Morse Peckham once labelled them (cited in Bate[7]), the 'directions for performance', the rules that, in our field, frame and shape what people in organisations do, and ultimately their and their users' experiences of the service they provide (think of the sequence: rules–behaviour–experience). The broad task of EBD in this regard is to surface and examine the design rules in the light of the patient experience and consider which of them may need to be changed or added.

Illustration 1: the 'immediate feedback' pattern/principle and the importance of 'entry' and 'exit' experiences

The *immediate feedback* design pattern or principle is a good illustration of how people's experiences of a product or service (especially the latter) may be deeply affected by whether or not this principle has been built into the design. There are two elements to this: what are called 'entry feedback' and 'exit feedback'. We switch on our computer or press the call button on the lift, and wait for the green light to come on or the up or down arrow to light up.[8] From an experience point of view it is crucial they do because it is the machine's only way of telling us: 'I heard you, I'm on my way.' Having received this almost instantaneous response to our initial (entry) action, whether this be auditory or visual responses or clues, we are then usually perfectly happy to wait until the computer boots up or the lift arrives, even if it takes some time for them to do this. Interestingly, at this early point, immediate feedback is more important than 'immediate service' – the service does not have to be instant to feel satisfactory or acceptable; for a while at least good feedback is the proxy for good service; we are happy to wait.

There are hundreds of such examples that underline the importance of the immediate feedback principle in the creation of positive human experiences, from the 'ticket' machine on the butcher's counter at the supermarket or post office that allows you to relax while you await your turn (and to know exactly where you are in the queuing process), to the WAIT sign on the pedestrian crossing that lights up when you press the 'cross' button, which may or may not have any controlling effect on the traffic lights; it doesn't really matter so long as you think it does. And just think what a difference it has made to be able to ring a company helpdesk and hear 'We have logged your call and you are number four in the queue' rather than 'All the lines are busy at the moment, please try again later' – yet another example of immediate and informed feedback that makes the wait tolerable and acceptable.

Now think of those occasions when the lift or computer light does not go on when you press it, the equivalent of not having the immediate feedback rule built into your design. What happens is you keep pressing it as if to say or implore, 'Where are you? When are you going to notice me?' You are lost and unhappy because you are unnoticed and helpless. Exactly the same applies when we go into a GP's surgery, A&E or any other hospital department. What we are looking for is clear and immediate feedback from the 'system' that flags up that our arrival has been noted ('Thank you, Mrs X, we have checked you in, now please take a seat'), that the 'machinery' has been activated, and that the service – the equivalent of the lift – is on its way. Unfortunately, this is not always the case: someone tells you to 'take a seat' and wait, or they check you in on a computer whose screen you can't see (similar to concealing the lift press button light!). There is no equivalent of a clear green light coming on. Watch people getting up from time to time in the waiting room, which is rarely to complain about the length of their wait but to inquire, 'You haven't forgotten me, have you? You do have me on your list?' In cases like these, feedback was not satisfactory at check-in, nor has it been during the wait itself.

The following extract from one NHS patient's story (cited in Bate[9]) shows just how important it is to build the immediate feedback principle into the design of a service – and what happens when it has not been. Patient B was a middle-aged male, complaining of severe groin pain.

> *Over the next week the pain got worse, and I was advised by a nurse at the local NHS walk-in centre to try the Accident & Emergency (A&E) department of our local hospital. Desperate for some relief, I decided to follow her advice. I went to A&E reception where there was someone seated behind some very thick glass (presumably for personal safety and security reasons) who said she could not properly hear me. She spoke back in a very thick foreign accent and I was embarrassed that I was unable to understand what she was saying and had to keep saying 'pardon'. This wasn't helped by her avoidance of any direct eye contact with me. Finally, I was able to deduce that I wasn't supposed to report to reception yet – if I had read the signs (and there were so many of them I had missed this one), I would have seen that I was supposed to take one of the 'pink' coloured seats in the main room and wait to be called by the medical staff.*
>
> *The problem was that all five of the pink seats were taken and there was no nurse in the booth in front of them to triage and put people in some kind of order. So I had to take a seat behind the pink seats which made me feel like I wasn't even checked-in – a bit like being at the supermarket fish counter and not having a ticket to say when your turn was. It had the effect of making me anxious because as far as I could see there was no queuing system and all the pink seats were taken. Other people came in and squeezed up next to me, looking equally anxious for the lack of formal check-in or attention. Two disembodied TVs hanging from the ceiling blasted out the same children's TV programme, and I noticed no-one was watching them. This wasn't surprising because the TVs were so high up they couldn't be seen from most of the seats, and many of them faced in the opposite direction. Finally the triage nurse appeared from behind and said 'who's next', at which point everyone stood up and said 'me'! A woman who had come in long after me went first . . .*

The key thing here is that people like Patient B want and expect immediate feedback just as they expect to wait, so in this sense, and somewhat ironically, it is the former that is the problem at this point not the latter (and perversely the more feedback they get, the more prepared they will be to wait). The question this therefore raises is why so much attention in healthcare has been given to the second and so little to the first, which may mean that waiting times go down a little for Patient B but his experience of the service has not significantly improved. We also need to add that feedback saves not wastes time, and is therefore good for efficiency and performance (P), not just quality (A), concerns. Most of it can be done technologically, thereby leaving nurses and staff to get on with their job, free of the endless inquiries and interruptions that stem from poor entry feedback. So, the point is simply that knowledge of this design principle by the hospital staff and improvement specialists might have led to a better service and a better patient experience.

In fact feedback is important at every stage of the journey, not just the beginning, and most healthcare systems are failing somewhere in this regard. A recent example was an outpatients department where we had been doing some EBD work with staff and patients. The staff had drawn our attention to the long waits for patients caused by overbookings, overruns, and delays looking for notes or awaiting test results: 'They seem to wait forever, but that's my perception' (staff nurse). Interestingly, patients did not seem to mind ('If someone overruns, it means their need is probably greater than mine. It could be me next time; I can wait'). However, what they did object to was not the delay *per se* but the lack of immediate feedback around it (*see* our lift example above). The delays 'whiteboard' in the reception area was clear indication, in theory at least, that notification of any delays would be relayed to patients immediately, which on the face of it was a very simple way of building the immediate feedback principle into the design of the service. However, the reality was somewhat different. For the first 40 minutes of the clinic on one of the days we sat in and observed it, the board remained blank, and then finally a nurse appeared and scribbled '40 minutes' on it before disappearing again (followed by a loud moan from those seated in the waiting area). Later, we asked, did it happen often that somebody omitted to put up the 10 minutes, 15 minutes delays and so on as the overruns accumulated, to which came the reply, 'Oh, yes, often, probably, because the nurses are around the other side trying to do other things like clean scopes and do whatever they're doing, and they do not have time to do the regular updates'. Whatever the justification, this was a very negative experience for patients because, as they pointed out to us, it meant that they were unable to leave the clinic even for a minute to grab a coffee or glass of water (dry throats being a particular problem for the patients being seen in this clinic) in case they missed their turn. Clear and immediate feedback with regular updates of the whiteboard would have made it a much more tolerable experience for all concerned.

Not only is it crucial to service design to observe the immediate feedback principle at the beginning of the episode, it is equally important that this happens at the end in exiting the system (the 'conclusion' phase of the experience) – the equivalent of the 'it is now safe to turn off your computer' alert. Patients and users need to be reassured that everything that needed to happen has happened, that the outcome has been successful, that knowledge of the experience has been safely saved, and that all the steps have been put in place to ensure that the follow-up process will automatically be triggered – not, as often happens, just to be told 'you can go now' or 'we'll be in touch' or 'someone will make contact with your GP at some point'. As Shedroff observes, a conclusion needs resolution:

> *The conclusion can come in many ways, but it must provide some sort of resolution . . . Often an experience that is engaging has no real end, leaving participants dissatisfied or even confused about the experience, emotions, or ideas they just felt.*[10]

In other words, ends do not just happen, in design they need to be *made* to happen; an ending has to be skilfully constructed. An important aspect to this is ensuring that the discharge is properly packaged, so that the patient leaves feeling better able to cope than when he or she came in. Sending a person off clutching various forms and medicines, accompanied by a bewildering list of instructions, is not likely to accomplish the experience of satisfactory termination of the care episode. The odd but informative example that interactive designers at IBM have used to underline the importance of satisfactory exit feedback in EBD is the dry cleaners:

> *When you pick up your clothes from the cleaners you see the clothes on their hangers, hear the rustling sound of their plastic sheaths, and feel their weight*

as you carry them. All these experiences serve feedback confirming that you suc-cessfully completed your errand.[8]

To sum up, this particular example of a design rule suggests that placing a similar focus in healthcare service design on instantaneous feedback at the beginning of the episode and properly completed feedback at the end might offer new insights into future services, and draw our attention to parts of the process that might otherwise be overlooked. Scoping work previously carried out by the NHS Modernisation Agency established that there are many other design rules and principles like these in the architecture and computing literatures that have the same or greater relevance to the design of healthcare services and patient experience.

Illustration 2: the rule of progressive disclosure

Human–computer interaction (HCI) designers talk about the importance of another design principle, this time in the design of computer software: the principle of *progressive disclosure*. Rather than put expert-level features at the same level as basic ones, and run the risk of confusing or overloading people, you put them behind a door marked 'expert', 'additional options' or 'advanced search':

> *Consider the car, where most folks can work with the controls in the cabin but, with a few exceptions (such as washer fluid) they never need to open the hood . . . A few experts do open it up and adjust the car with these expert-level controls, and if you want to do it, you know where to look. But if operating a car presented you with the entire engine as a control structure, most humans would find driving dauntingly complex, even if they just had to learn not to look at 'all them wires and tubes and valves and things.'*[11]

Unlikely as it may appear, this principle is relevant to the healthcare setting in a number of ways. Take hospital signage. It is a well-established fact, and the source of some jocularity, that patients and visitors are always getting lost in a hospital, the main reason being that they are confronted by far too much of the information on a wall to be able to digest 'in one go' (and not helped by the fact that a lot of it is in medical-speak). There is information overload. Progressive disclosure, on the other hand, would begin a thinning-out process by taking out the specialist signposts that are only relevant to staff (e.g. Pathology lab) and that do not need to be put on public display (as in the case of our computer desktop). Additionally, like a motorway or road system, rather than signpost every road from John O' Groats to Land's End on one huge sign, the hospital signage would aim to give you the bare minimum to get you to the next 'turn off', and then reveal further directions to you as you go (the equivalent of 'outpatients follow signs for Barnsley and the north', followed by ever more destination-targeted information) – the notion of progressive disclosure.

The progressive disclosure principle is also relevant at the microsystem level of a healthcare organisation, especially at key points where ensuring the patient–staff interaction is right is absolutely crucial. For example, one key issue (which we discuss in more detail in Chapter 9) in our own co-design work with head and neck cancer patients is how the bad news gets broken to the newly diagnosed cancer sufferer. The surgeon and oncologist have to decide how much information to give, at what pace and in what form. Some patients, like the equivalent of our car fanatics or computer buffs, may want it all, in one go, but that is rare. Clinical staff were well aware that a patient in shock or denial takes in little if anything at all at that first meeting; for example, all that one head and neck cancer patient could remember of her experience of being told that she had cancer was that she would now be able to receive free aromatherapy treatments!

> *You know you're talking to a patient and they're just completely, the glazed look comes over their eyes and you just think, it's not the right time to go through this. We need to support the patient, we need to bring them back if that's the best thing to do but when they leave the clinic they must, must, must have [the clinical nurse specialist's] contact number, we must make sure the GP knows what's happened, they must have a support network in the community because that's a big time for them, when they leave the clinic and they may have to wait another week before they see us and what are they thinking that whole time? What's going through their mind, they probably think 'I am dying', I'm sure that's what nearly all of them think. 'I am dying, right now'.*
> (Surgeon 1)

The design principle for this interaction and process is therefore one of progressive disclosure: tell patients only what they want or need to know at that point in time, and space out the interaction and disclosure over a series of meetings, letting them set and guide the level, detail and pace of information disclosure relating to their condition.

As the following quotation from another surgeon shows, although they don't actually use the words 'progressive disclosure', this 'principle' is very much part of their 'theory-in-use', and frames many of the tough calls and judgements they have to make:

> *You do it [break the bad news] by judging the situation with the person you are talking to and try to judge where they want you to place it and where you had better place it. The first time I see them I sort of introduce them to the idea that this could be cancer and the next time I see them I confirm that. So, you take them through different stages and different parts of their journey.*
> (Surgeon 2)

Reframed as 'progressive disclosure,' the issue shifts the design challenge from the more usual 'communication' to 'information management' – the how and the how much rather than the what. Disclose too fast for the patient to take in (i.e. absorb and assimilate) and there will be dysfunction and a very uncomfortable and stressful experience ('can't take in/can't process/can't make sense'; for example, carers told us how their partners sometimes refused to read the information booklets they were given because there was too much information for them to take in 'in one go', which is why they, the carers, often found themselves drawn into the information management process, reading and filtering information back to their partners). On the other hand, disclose too slowly and the patient may see you as 'keeping something back' or not 'levelling' or being straight with the patient about their condition. Evidence that the pacing is about right will ultimately come in the form of the patient actually asking for more information about their illness, a process that begins to look more and more like co-management of the information surrounding the condition, and ultimately leading to a patient who is an 'expert' in their condition.

The design organisation IDEO gives other examples of design rules or principles for health care which, like the above, seem incontrovertible and even universal in their appeal. These include:[12]

- privacy anywhere, anytime
- make the opaque transparent
- patients and families never wait
- patients own the experience.

We therefore believe that at both the macro and micro levels of healthcare there is arguably as strong a case for service designers to become aware of the design rules upon which the service is designed as there is for an industrial designer to know the design rules for a building or a product. After all, it is only through knowing what these are that we can begin to learn and construct new and better rules and better practices and experiences. Take the example of design rules for new digital products: designers have begun to come up with design rules that look very different from the traditional ones – for example, 'open-ended', 'social and user-controlled', 'robust and forgiving', 'physical and sensory', 'flexible and personal'.[13] Not that healthcare services necessarily require the same ones (although having a service that is social and personal does have immediate relevance and appeal), but rather it needs to search for and then nurture its own.

Good and bad common sense (patterns and anti-patterns)

It is often overlooked that such patterns and rules as we have described are cultural phenomena, part of the taken-for-granted 'common sense' of the organisation (literally *common*, shared or collective sense or meaning) and therefore that any change of patterns is likely to be accompanied not only by changes in behaviour and practice, but also by some kind of cultural shift – the notion of design as cultural change. Trice and Beyer write: 'People tell one another stories all the time; they become cultural forms when they are widely shared and come to carry distinct cultural meanings.'[14] Legends and sagas 'like stories, are actually celebrated parts of the organisational culture that are told and retold to new members and others to explain the organisation'.[14] The added bonus of focusing on design rules in the design process, therefore, is that changes in those rules are interventions that may well lead to important changes in the culture of an organisation or microsystem. But there are dangers.

Despite society's preference for regarding common sense as good – even superior – sense (often paying it the highest compliment by calling it 'conventional *wisdom*'), there can be 'good' common sense and 'bad' common sense, even 'nonsense' common sense! Appearances can be deceptive. The task for the designer is to get behind the common sense–good sense appearance of a design rule – whether this be an existing one or one that has been agreed for the future – and ask, is it really a good design rule? (Remember it was once common sense that told us the world was flat.) Framed in the language of the patterns designer, he or she needs to establish whether it is a 'design pattern' or an 'anti-pattern'.

Whereas a design pattern is a 'good' and sensible rule or principle to follow (for us the immediate feedback rule described above would be an example of this), an anti-pattern is a 'bad' design rule posing as a good one. On the surface, an anti-pattern appears to be sensible, correct and functional but is in fact a design flaw or mistake that may wreak havoc with the design, whether it be something like a computer, change programme or a diabetes service. In fact what happens if the anti-pattern goes undetected is that failure is literally programmed into the design, and nothing can be done to rescue it, short of removing the guilty assumption or piece of logic and starting again. Here we therefore have a classic case of an attempted or intended solution that has become the problem itself.[15]

'Anti-patterns' are currently mainly confined to the domain of computer science and software design but we would argue strongly that they have huge, as yet mostly unexplored, potential for the domains of the social, management and organisational sciences. For example, we would argue strongly that many change and improvement projects don't *go wrong*; they went wrong *even before they started* as a result of flawed or false assumptions, rules or logic being 'programmed' into the design.

An example: 'scaling fallacy'

In the design sciences, such as architecture and engineering, one familiar anti-pattern, which a change or improvement programme also needs to be on guard against, is known as the 'scaling fallacy'.[4] This is the tendency to assume that a system that works at one scale will also work at a smaller or larger scale (also known as cube law and law of sizes). Put more simply, just because something works at one level, that does not necessarily mean it will work above or below that level. The compelling example often used is the magic of flying (*see* Figure 7.1). To illustrate, starting and then moving up from the bottom, aeroplankton float (but do not fly), baby spiders use web sails to parachute (but do not fly), insects flap to fly (and some can fly), birds flap to fly (and do fly), humans flap . . . but do not fly! At very small and very large scales, flapping to fly is not a viable strategy, because at a small scale the wings are too small to displace air molecules, and at very large scales the effects of gravity are too great for flapping to work.

By the same token, change models and designs can be effective at one scale and completely ineffective at another, and just because they work at, say, a small project level (e.g. in a hospital department), this does not mean they will 'fly' at a higher level, across an entire organisation or healthcare system. As Bevan and Plsek have thus argued:

> Most improvement projects cannot be scaled up in a linear way to go from pilots to transformation of the whole system. Large system change requires connected action at every level of the system; and it is the complexity of the interconnections that defies simple scaling.[16]

Nor is it simply a case of putting more effort in to making your change programme 'fly'. No matter how much faster you flap, you are sadly never going to take off. Humans flying calls for different design rules from those of birds – which is roughly where the story of aviation begins.

Pressman and Wildavsky use a similar metaphor to drive home the same point:

> Biologists tell us that embryonic tissue of the fruit fly Drosophila is capable of developing into a wing, a leg, or an antenna, according to the influences brought to bear on it. Also, the tissues of the flank of a newt are capable of developing into a leg, but it would be impossible to induce a fish to develop a leg, or a horse to develop a wing. Whereas policies can assume marvellous new

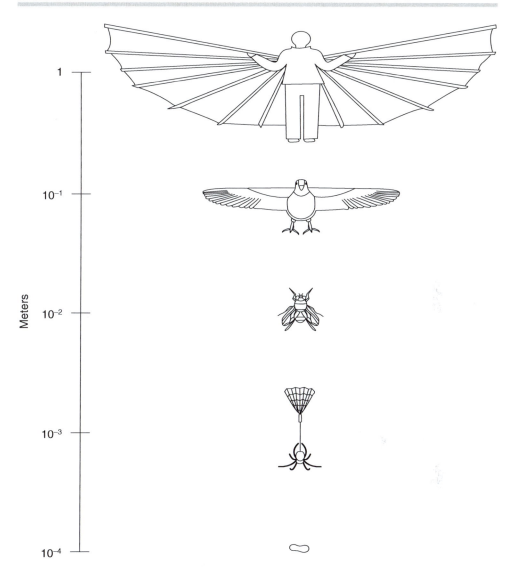

Figure 7.1 The scaling fallacy. *Source:* Lidwell *et al.*[4]

forms during implementation, in order to understand policy evolution (or indeed any type of evolution), it is as important to understand what cannot happen as what can.[17]

Sadly, old assumptions (and theories) die hard, and once the wrong assumptions have been programmed in, people are generally reluctant to backtrack on these. No-one likes to have their assumptions challenged or admit they were wrong in the first place; in fact the opposite may occur and they may become even more wedded to them. Organisation theorists refer to this as the escalation of commitment to a failing course of action! An example of this surfaced in one government minister's comment several years ago about the NHS modernisation programme: 'Programmes are getting results, so what we therefore need are more programmes', an approach which only now is being replaced by new approaches and new design principles for large-scale change.

Stop following the wrong rules

Identifying anti-patterns (what does not work but looks like it does work) can be as important to design as identifying patterns (what does work), since the second is about guidelines to follow and the first about guidelines that are being followed that should perhaps stop being followed – negative solutions that present more problems than they address. Identification and investigation of previously undetected anti-patterns provides the knowledge to prevent or recover from them. An example of an anti-pattern we discuss later is the notion of 'always tell the patient what the next steps are', which on the face of it seems like a very good – and sound common sense – design principle but which may, in some circumstances, provide the patient with such a daunting view of what is to come that they lose the will to proceed with the treatment. In this example, the good sense becomes bad sense because it takes away resilience from the patients.

That is the problem with anti-patterns: they seem so *irrefutable* and *right* – such perfect common sense! For example, how could one possibly argue with IDEO's 'privacy anywhere, anytime' design principle? Well Patient B, for one, might want to:

> *My first impressions of the Treatment Centre (TC) were so much better than anything I had experienced before. A lovely refurbished building, and a single en-suite room. It was only later I was to discover that there were downsides to the TC and that it certainly was not the place to be when things go wrong. The doors has such strong springs on them that they could not even be propped open, hence the door was always closed and you were completely isolated. There was a small glass panel through which you could be observed – a bit like Cell Block H – made even smaller by the fact that your file was clipped on to it on the outside. There was a bracket fitting in the room for a TV – from a time, I was told, when this was a private ward – but I had been told that no-one had been prepared to invest in TVs. So there were no people, no TV, no radio, only bare white walls. There was no day room either where one could meet with other patients. Least conspicuous of all were the clinicians – I was told they didn't like the TC and treated it like a satellite country. I didn't realise until then that a 'nurse-led service' actually meant a 'clinician absent service'. (Recorded story of Patient B, November 2004)*

So it is that the experience of privacy can actually sometimes be one of isolation and loneliness, whether this be for a patient like Patient B, or an old person (a familiar story) who, having been given a private room, asks to go back on the general ward where she can have more people to talk to.

These last two examples show how situation- and person-specific design patterns in an organisational context really are. This is what makes designing in a social setting so much more difficult than designing in a technical setting, since what may be a 'good' design pattern for one kind of customer or one kind of situation may turn out to be a 'bad' anti-pattern for another (reinforcing the case for developing different user personas and carrying out a rigorous 'contextual inquiry' – *see* pages 84–5). It also suggests that perhaps the most valuable aspect of thinking 'design rules' lies not in treating them as universal and inviolable truths, but in setting them up as polarities,[18] so that the upsides and downsides of both can be considered and debated, and proper (and often subtle and difficult) judgements and decisions sensibly and intelligently made, including where and when it might be sensible to depart from them.

Difficulties and reservations apart, design patterns (good and bad) do help us to become aware of, understand and explain the *current* situation and how it is put together – both why and how it works (Buckminster Fuller's 'know why' as cited in Kleiner[19]) but also why it is not working or working as well as it should (the all-too-common scenario in change management programmes of 'underachievement' – the implementation gap between ambition and outcome). But, further to that, design patterns may also help us begin to explore, and ultimately test out, what might become a new design concept for the *future* – a potential design solution. This is a point we take up in the case study in Chapter 9, revealing one of the great advantages of the EBD process that design patterns may be created, and anti-patterns weeded out, by staff and patients in partnership.

It is interesting to note in passing that, while design patterns do not figure explicitly in organisational research, even despite the strong current interest in design and design sciences, they remain implicit in the approach. For example, Gephart[20] writes that 'an important challenge for qualitative research is to articulate rules or bases for deciding "associations"'. There is the 'how' question as well as the 'what' question to be considered here. One useful way of thinking about how a service or process should be configured may be to use the metaphor of patterns as (to borrow a phrase from Robert Pirsig's *Zen and the Art of Motorcycle Maintenance*[21]) signposting the many 'paths there are up the mountain', and anti-patterns as the many 'paths to disaster'[15] (a kind of snakes and ladders of design).

Counter-narratives

One final note that links back to our earlier chapter on stories and storytelling is that, just as narrative can be a powerful way of identifying past and present design rules and patterns, so can counter-narrative be an equally powerful way of constructing future design patterns and designs themselves. Buckler and Zein[22] talk about 'maverick stories' giving users a licence to break rules, and this is literally what one is also able to achieve in the case of design rules. Elsewhere, one of us has described how a multidisciplinary healthcare team effectively engaged in developing and acting out various counter-narratives around service improvement, using such stories to highlight the failures of the service and stigmatise the organisation culture that caused these, and in so doing putting the case for radical counter-cultural change. In the process of telling stories 'against' the negative aspects of the current service, those involved were able to construct a 'from-to' map for change, and agree 'rule changes' that would allow the transition to occur.[23,24]

References

1 Gamma E, Helm R, Johnson R *et al*. *Design Patterns: Elements of Reusable Object-Oriented Software*. New York: Addison-Wesley; 1995.
2 Alexander C. *A Pattern Language*. Oxford: Oxford University Press; 1977.

3 Alexander C. *The Timeless Way of Building*. Oxford: Oxford University Press Press; 1979.

4 Lidwell W, Holden K, Butler J. *Principles of Design, 100 Ways to Enhance Usability, Influence Perception, Increase Appeal, and Make Better Design Decisions*. Gloucester, MA; Rockport; 2003.

5 Romme AGL, Endenburg G. Construction principles and design rules in the case of circular design. *Organisation Science*. 2006; **17**(2): 287–97.

6 Plsek P, Bibby J and Whitby E. Design rules grounded in the experience of managers: a system for organizational learning and pilot study of practical methods. *Journal of Applied Behavioral Science*. 2007; **43**(1): 153–70.

7 Bate SP. *Strategies for Cultural Change*. Oxford: Butterworth-Heinemann; 1995.

8 IBM. Ease of use – what is user experience design? 2005. www-03.ibm.com/easy/page/2 (accessed 7 December 2006).

9 Bate SP. Ethnography with 'attitude': mobilising narratives for public sector change. In: Veenswijk M, editor. *Organising Innovation. New Approaches to Cultural Change and Intervention in Public Sector Organisations*. Amsterdam: IOS Press; 2006. p. 105–32.

10 Shedroff N. Experience design. www.webreference.com/authoring/design/expdesign/index.html (accessed 3 August 2006).

11 Arnold K. Programmers are people, too. *Security*. 2005; **3**(5). www.acmqueue.com/modules.php?name=Content&pa=printer_friendly&pid=3 (accessed 30 August 2005).

12 Leighton Heart and Vascular Center for Memorial Hospital and Health System. Patient-centered care experience. www.ideo.com/portfolio/re.asp?x=50185 (accessed 12 August 2004).

13 Mäkelä A, Fulton Suri J. Supporting users' creativity: design to induce pleasurable experiences. *Proceedings of the Conference on Affective Human Factors*. London: Asean Academic Press; 2001. p. 387–91.

14 Trice HM, Beyer JM. *The Cultures of Work Organisations*. Englewood Cliffs, NJ: Prentice Hall; 1993.

15 Brown WH, Malveau RC, McCormick HW *et al*. *Antipatterns. Refactoring Software, Architectures, and Projects in Crisis*. Chichester: Wiley; 1998.

16 Bevan H, Plsek P. *Toward a Model for Making Modernisation Mainstream*. Unpublished working paper; 2002.

17 Pressman JL, Wildavsky A. *Implementation*. Berkeley, CA; University of Southern California Press; 1984. p. 173.

18 Johnson B. *Polarity Management: Identifying and Managing Unsolvable Problems*. Amherst, MA: HRD Press; 1996.

19 Kleiner A. *The Age of Heretics. Heroes, Outlaws and the Forerunners of Corporate Change*. London: Nicholas Brearley; 1996.

20 Gephart RP. Qualitative research and the Academy of Management Journal. *Academy of Management Journal*. 2004; **47**(4): 456.

21 Pirsig RM. *Zen and the Art of Motorcycle Maintenance*. London: The Bodley Head; 1974.

22 Buckler SA, Zein KA. From experience: the spirituality of innovation: learning from stories. *Journal of Production Innovation Management*. 1996; **13**: 391–405.

23 Bate SP. The role of stories and storytelling in organisational change efforts: the anthropology of an intervention in a UK hospital. *Intervention. Journal of Culture, Organisation and Management*. 2004; **1**(1): 27–42.

24 Bate SP. The role of stories and storytelling in organisational change efforts: a field study of an emerging community of practice within the UK National Health Service. In: Hurwitz B, Greenhalgh T, Skultans V, editors. *Narrative Research in Health and Illness*. London: BMJ Publications; 2004. p. 325–48.

Chapter 8

Experience-based design: tools for diagnosis and intervention

So you must learn to think like your user. (Ken Arnold)

One of the design profession's major strengths is the ability to create tangible and often very user-friendly methods for the expression of ideas, to exploit new tools, and pragmatically adapt existing ones for the task in hand.[1] As we have suggested – although they have been appropriated by the design professions, especially experience and interactive design, and have indeed been found to work extremely well together[2,3] – a number of the methods central to an EBD process began their lives in ethnography not design. It is important to remember, however, that while EBD uses a number of ethnographic methods (adding up to what Van Maanen would collectively term 'fieldwork') it is not the aim of EBD to write ethnographies, which is a different activity altogether. Rather, ethnographic-based methods and tools, individually or in combination, may be called into service purely to gain access to, and design, user experiences. For this reason it is possible to allay anxieties, often heard expressed, that in-depth, ethnographic inquiry 'takes too long' (the perfect excuse for skipping research and diagnosis altogether). Although this may be the case in an ethnographic or anthropological setting, in a design setting, design professionals have shown that it is quite possible to adapt ethnographic methods for short-term projects, for example by focusing tightly on key issues rather than trying to gain an overview of the whole situation.[4]

What follows is a brief review of some of the methods one may find in experience-based and participatory design, ranging from those that require only marginal involvement from users, to others that demand their full-blown participation. This is only a small sample from a huge selection. For example, Muller describes over 60 different methods in participative design practice alone.[5] We have divided the methods and tools into (a) diagnostic methods, and (b) intervention methods, although both may be combined in the actual EBD process. The chapter then concludes with a presentation and discussion of an intriguing case study from the United States of how methods for designing the physical environment can be integrated with those for designing experiences.

Diagnostic methods

Using informants

In the early days of an EBD project, putting together a representative sample of people to interview may be less pressing than finding key *informants*, people who can introduce or induct the researcher-designer into the organisation or microsystem under study, and act as one's guide to the best people and places to begin one's search for 'experience'. Millen suggests that such guides should be 'people with access to a broad range of people and activities and be able to discuss in advance where interesting behaviours are most likely to be observed'.[6] In the particular case of EBD in healthcare, one is often looking for staff who not only know which of their colleagues the researcher(s) should be put in touch with, but also which patients and carers might make good informants or interviewees. One recent example of this expert guide in our work was a clinical nurse practitioner around whom the whole department was found to revolve, but who also played a key liaison role with patients in the clinic and at home and knew them intimately. She was strategically so well placed as to be able to point us in the direction of patients and staff, some of the latter quite marginal to the microsystem but nevertheless brilliant as commentators on the whole work scene. She was also in her own right a goldmine of information on the staff experience of giving care and the patient experience of receiving it.

Contextual inquiry

Using key informants and guides to help do a preliminary 'reccy' of the area is only part of the bigger activity of carrying out a thoroughgoing 'contextual inquiry'.[7–10] In a contextual inquiry:

> an experienced interviewer observes users in the context of their actual work situation, performing their usual job tasks ... Conducting a contextual inquiry normally involves a team of two, an inquirer and a note-taker/observer. The inquirer and the participant are equals; each is an expert in his or her own work. After the visits, the inquiry team reviews their notes and analyses the information to find patterns, often using affinity diagrams. Contextual inquiries yield rich data from seeing users in their real work context, and thus can identify issues not previously recognised.[11]

For an illustration of the method and value of contextual inquiry in a contemporary healthcare setting we refer readers to the case study description in Chapter 9. We also refer them back to Chapter 7 on design patterns where we made the point that contextual inquiry is especially necessary given how situation-specific organisation design patterns will be.

According to Raven and Flanders,[10] contextual inquiry is based on the following three principles:

- data gathering must take place in the context of the users' work
- the data gatherer and the user form a partnership to explore issues together
- the inquiry is based on a focus; that is, it is based on a clearly defined set of concerns, rather than a list of specific questions (as in a survey).

Contextual inquiry is necessary for two reasons: first, because meaning and action can only be rendered intelligible in relation to the context within which they occur, indeed are shaped by it ('context' being the commonplace, familiar and everyday world within which people live); second, because one important consequence of doing contextual inquiry is that the designer is able to help people begin to 'see the familiar in unfamiliar ways':

> [Designers] look at what is commonplace and familiar, and they reveal the ways in which it is unique, allowing them to break through existing assumptions and acceptance of things as 'the way it's always been done' so that new opportunities for change can be explored.[12]

Contextual inquiry has also started to make inroads into the electronic and cyber context of organisations. For example (*see* conversational archive later), being given access to a person's email now makes it possible for designers to gain a deep understanding of the work context within which that person's communicative practices are situated and embedded.

Ethnographic interviewing[13,14]

As the root discipline for EBD, anthropology – not surprisingly – also furnishes it with its core methods, which are mostly qualitative, unstructured, participant observational, informal and conversational (from the Latin meaning 'wandering together with'), the dominant metaphor being researcher as traveller (coming back with a story to tell), rather than researcher as miner (coming back with the buried treasure).[14] Van Maanen makes the same distinction in the following way:

> *Fieldwork is not of an ethnographic sort when it is pursued by a team of social researchers on a sort of expedition or Foucault-like panopticon observation-and-interview project. Fieldwork of an ethnographic kind is authentic to the degree it approximates the stranger stepping into a culturally alien community to become, for a time and in an unpredictable way, an active part of the face-to-face relationships in that community.*[15]

Anschuetz and Rosenbaum describe in simple, straightforward terms what ethnographic interviewing is, at the same time going some way towards demystifying it:

> *Ethnographic interviewing uses techniques from anthropology to collect concrete information from people in their context of use. Sessions are conducted in work or home environments, where people behave more naturally and where we can explore surroundings and artefacts to add validity to self-reported data. Ethnographic interviews are useful for learning about the needs, work processes, and preferences of target audiences ...*[4]

Equally helpfully, Heyl[16] provides an overview of the huge literature that deals with this method, beginning with the goals of ethnographic interviewing, an activity that follows on from the initial induction into the culture and its people:

- listen well and respectfully, developing an ethical engagement with the participants at all stages of the project
- acquire a self-awareness of your role in the construction of meaning during the interview process (co-construction)
- be cognisant of the ways in which both the ongoing relationship and the broader social context affect the participants, the interview process, and the project outcomes
- recognise that dialogue is discovery and only partial knowledge will ever be attained.

To which we may add:

- pose open-ended questions of the 'Tell me what you know about ...', 'What was the best time ...?', 'What is the funniest thing that has happened?' variety. Signal where you want the discussion to go but always give the speaker the opportunity to take it somewhere else.

Interviews are first and foremost interaction; a conversation between the researcher and the interviewee in which they quite literally swap and explore 'world views'. Citing Kvale,[14] Heyl identifies seven stages of an interview investigation:[17]

- thematising (researcher thinks through primary goals and questions)
- designing
- interviewing
- transcribing
- analysing
- verifying
- reporting.

Interviewing can take place anywhere – the workplace, the home, the place where the experience is or has taken place[9] – the best guide being to take the project out to wherever people are using or contemplating using the service. As already noted, it is generally recognised that the best and most effective way of eliciting information is to use open-ended questions such as: 'Have you used this service before?', 'What do you remember most about what happened?', 'Did you like it the way it was?', 'What things were missing?', 'Why not tell us your story from the beginning?'

Discovery Interviews

A commonly used approach to interviewing patients and carers in the healthcare service improvement field is that of the Discovery Interview. The Discovery Interview (DI) is defined as:

> ... an innovative technique designed to 'improve care by understanding patient and carer experiences better and by gaining insight into their needs'.[18] They are based upon a philosophy that puts patients and carers at the centre, and values listening to their experiences as a way of gaining insight into their needs which is unavailable elsewhere.[17]

As Figure A (*see* Appendix, page 116) shows, the DI is extremely well thought through as a method, consisting of three types of activity that the discovery team work through in order, namely: preparation, interviewing, and implementation.

It is quite evident from Figure A that many of the features of a DI (unstructured but with a 'spine' of questions based on the stages of a patient's journey; narrative and story-based; tape-recorded and transcribed; shared with clinical teams; the identification of issues/areas for service improvement) and the discovery process itself are the same or very similar to those we have just described under the heading of ethnographic interviewing, as well as the EBD process more generally. However, the big difference between DIs and an EBD process is best highlighted by one of the key findings of a recent evaluation of a DI approach in a collaborative programme to improve services for coronary heart disease patients in the NHS:

> During all the data-collection exercises undertaken as part of this project, the strongest message to emerge was that not all discovery interview teams had reached the stage of sharing stories with clinical teams and achieving service

improvements ... this is the most difficult aspect of the technique, relying as it does on the engagement of highly pressurised, highly trained staff who may not be open to hearing what may be perceived as anecdotal criticisms of their work.[18]

In short, the connection between story, service design and action/improvement may actually end up being quite weak. The findings from the evaluation in question is that while staff were clearly moved by the stories they heard, and their attitudes towards patients did change as a result, there were still more than half of them who admitted that there had been no change in their everyday behaviour or actions. The evaluation concluded: 'This appears to suggest that DIs have a greater power to change people's perceptions of patients and carers on an individual basis than to lead to individual changes in behaviour'. More worrying, the majority of those interviewed felt that there had been no changes in departmental level (55%) or clinical team level (68%) care, services or facilities as a result of the DI process. Furthermore, and in a similar vein, 62% of the respondents felt that DIs had had no impact on the use or structure of care pathways.

What are we to conclude from this? Undoubtedly, DIs do perhaps come closest to the essence of EBD than any other technique currently in use in healthcare, and could quite easily become an integral part of any EBD project with some minor modification. However, it is the additional work that EBD entails with regard to it also being an OD process that directly engages patients as well as staff (not just the discovery team but a large number of other staff as well) in the design process from stories, through joint analysis and interpretation to implementation that distinguishes EBD from DIs alone. This distinction is an important one in terms of resolving the dilemma in the quotation above, and the disappointing results revealed by the evaluation, while at the same reinforcing the comment we made earlier that stories in themselves do not bring about change: stories may mobilise and energise a change/design process but it is the change process itself and the direct and active participation of staff and patients in it that produces implementation and action, and ultimately spread and sustainability.

The criticism that can therefore be levelled at DIs in their present form, and, arguably, narrative and patient voices programmes more widely (*see*, for example, www.dipex.org and www.patientvoices.org.uk), is that the stories (especially website ones) are too often stand-alone and not connected to any kind of organisational development or service improvement process. People, including patients, may learn from them, indeed be moved by them, but this in itself may not connect to any kind of service improvement process or activity. As it is presently constituted, the DI process is also somewhat exclusive as an activity, being focused on the work of a core DI team, who gather and interpret the stories, and lead the Plan, Do, Study, Act process, with only minimal involvement from patients (in the shape of add-on 'focus groups'). Unlike EBD there is no co-design with patients and staff at every stage of the process, and no scope for joint analysis and interpretation of the stories they have told. In the DI process, patients are effectively reduced to playing the bit-part role of 'stories donors', who, having given up their experiences to the Discovery team, are then sent on their way, taking no further part in the design process.

Based on this critique, the way forward for DI in future does seem quite obvious, to us at least: begin to open up the process by populating each stage of the DI diagram in Figure A with patients and a wider group of staff, and replace the (staff/specialist only) Discovery team with the kind of co-design group (staff, patients, service improvement specialists) that will be described in our next chapter.

Participant and user interactive observation[19,20]

Anthropology also attaches great importance to directly observing people in their natural work habitat, not only talking to them but simply watching them, the value of this being able to see how they go about their everyday business in real time. Just sitting in, say, an outpatients department, and watching the comings and goings of patients and staff, their behaviour, interactions and the scripts they use to deal with each other, is invariably rewarded with rich insight into how and why things work, and how they might ultimately be redesigned for the better. What we have found surprising in this regard is how patients and outsiders like ourselves may see one thing and internal staff another.

For example, in one clinic we observed, patients were often confused by the requirement for them to queue up behind a red line painted on the floor before being called forward to be checked in for their appointment by the receptionist (a practice similar to that found in many hotels today). The problem was that some did not notice the line on entering, and proceeded to walked straight up to the desk – only to be sent to the back of the queue by the receptionist in full view of the rest of the queue of people. And not only did the line create embarrassment for those who missed it, it also caused frustration and irritation to those who had seen it, and were patiently waiting their turn. Such a procedure had been introduced after it had been discovered by a visiting review team some years earlier that patients were not being given sufficient privacy during their check-in. However, it required only a few minutes in the clinic for us to realise that, even with the new arrangement, every word of the exchange between receptionist and patient could be clearly heard by everyone seated in the waiting area! The line also had symbolic portent for patients: 'I would think that once you're over that line you move into the institutional side, as it were. If you stand on this side, you're a client, you're a person. If you go over that line then you are the property of the hospital' (patient).

Apart from being a touch point in its own right (and later to receive the full attention of the EBD team), the interesting thing is that when we raised the issue of the line with the lead surgeon in the clinic, he asked 'What line?', adding, 'I didn't know there was such a line until you just mentioned it.' Similar issues came up with the weighing scales in the clinic which, being located in a narrow corridor, caused considerable difficulty for old or obese patients as they struggled in the confined space to take off their shoes and climb onto them. In this case, the surgeon had to ask where the scales were, again not having previously noticed them. We revisit this particular 'touch point' in Chapter 9; it is used here to further illustrate the value of observational data. The other point to note is that just because something like a red line or set of weighing scales is small and mundane, or even (to some at least) trivial, this does not necessarily mean that it is insignificant. The whole point about 'touch points' is that they may figure strongly in people's emotions but not even register on the staff dials.

The proper name for this element of the initial research activity is participant observation,[21,22] but we prefer just to call it 'organisational loitering'. (Van

Maanen comments that the phrase 'participant observation' is 'less a definition for a method than it is an amorphous representation of the researcher's situation during a study'!) Observers may 'silently' loiter in a variety of different ways: by just sitting around and watching or writing notes, drawing diagrams and pictures (e.g. interactional maps) or using check-off lists (for example Bales' group behaviours inventory). With the opportunities offered by today's portable video cameras, researchers might more actively loiter by offering to do a video walkthrough with staff (as we did in the case study – *see* Chapter 9), patients and carers, asking them to point out and comment on various aspects of the physical or social environment, and generally providing a second 'pair of eyes' for this observational aspect of the work. Kuniavsky calls this joint activity, be it with staff or patients, 'user interactive observation':

> *This requires going to where people are engaged in the kind of activity the experience for which you are designing, and asking them to teach you about their activities. Most of the time should be spent observing what the participants are doing, what tools they are using, and how they are using them.*[20]

This is also where the apprentice role described earlier comes in:

> *One effective technique is to take on the role of an apprentice and asking them to give a running description of what they are doing. As in an expert-apprentice relationship, this should be enough to describe the practice to the apprentice, but not enough to interrupt the flow of the work. As an apprentice, you may occasionally ask for explanations, clarifications, or walkthroughs of actions, but do not let it drive the discussion.*[20]

A specific technique for observing people – and one we employed in the case study (Chapter 9) – is shadowing:

> *Shadowing is a research technique which involves a researcher closely following a member of an organisation over an extended period of time. When the person being shadowed goes to another department, the researcher follows them. When they have a project meeting or meet with a customer, the researcher sits in. If they have a coffee with friends who are colleagues from another site, the researcher goes too ... Throughout the shadowing period the researcher asks questions which will prompt a running commentary from the person being shadowed ... during the shadowing the researcher will write an almost continuous set of field notes ... at the end of the shadowing period the researcher will have a rich, dense and comprehensive data set which gives a detailed, first-hand and multi-dimensional picture of the role, approach, philosophy and tasks of the person being studied.*[23]

McDonald reviewed the literature on shadowing as a qualitative research technique to 'reveal the subtleties of perspective and purpose shaping those actions in the real-time context of an organisation'.[23] Her review article also provides practical recommendations for shadowers as well as discussing some of the problems with the technique. Shadowing can be used for (a) experiential learning, (b) as a means of recording behaviour, and (c) as a means of understanding roles or perspectives. It is a combination of the latter two purposes in which we are most interested from an EBD perspective.

Photographs

Designers will often take and hang up photographs of people they have met or places they have been to keep these in their mind's eye as they design. Similar photos may be displayed of physical buildings, equipment, gardens and so on in order to provide an ambient environment for design.

There is an equally strong tradition in anthropology and ethnography of using photographs as sources of data.[22] Van Maanen cites two studies that demonstrate the evocative power of still photography.[24] In the EBD case study we describe in Chapter 9 we used photography mainly as a means of recording our process; that then allowed us to share that process with a wider audience (for example, to update staff on progress with the project and to disseminate our work in other organisations), although patients participating in the study were also given disposable 'camera packs' to take away and record their experiences.

As we shall discuss later, photographs and video can be much more than a visual record for the diagnostic phase of a service improvement process. They can also play a decisive role in the intervention itself. Readers familiar with Zana Briski and Ross Kauffman's recent prize-winning documentary on the children of prostitutes in Calcutta, *Born Into Brothels*, in which the kids were taught how to use cameras to record their everyday life, will know how powerful such images can be in moving one to take action to improve people's lives – the notion of 'mobilising images', images that provide the energy and inspiration for people to make change, that make change an imperative. Mobilising images and mobilising narratives (*see* later) together are really what make EBD the powerful kind of intervention we know it can be.

Storytelling (and critical incidents[25])

We refer readers back to Chapter 6 on storytelling as a tool for gathering information on experience. The storyteller is more powerful than the interviewee, in the sense that he or she is guiding and controlling the interaction, rather than merely responding to someone else's questions. The structure and order is theirs not the interviewer's. Currently we tend to ask patients to tell us about their care and they do so telling us whatever information they choose to select. Narrative-based, storytelling methodologies[26] can be used to evoke responses as naturally and easily as possible. These are roughly based upon a chronological reconstruction of what happened – the story – with minimal 'prompting' intervention from the researchers (who? what? when? what happened next? etc.). As patients tell their stories along the time-line, researchers stop them from time to time to explore a particular 'touch point' in more detail ('So how did that feel? What was/would have been more helpful, satisfactory, less surprising/upsetting?') before returning to the unfolding narrative.

One very exciting recent development with huge potential for service design has been storytelling by 'blog', in which people have used the internet to share their stories with others and to keep in touch by means of a daily diary. Because computers and the internet are so much more accessible to the younger generation, one real gain is that this new technology has opened up new ways of giving voice to sick children, especially those with serious illness who have been isolated from other children because of that illness. Even as we write, a national television news channel has been running a feature on eight-year-old leukaemia sufferer Sophie Foxley whose story first appeared in her local newspaper after she began writing a blog charting her battle with the illness, and the loss of her hair during chemotherapy. The article was headed 'Brave Sophie's story goes online'.[27]

> *An eight-year-old Shrewsbury girl who is battling with leukaemia is keeping an online diary so her friends can stay in touch with her progress and send her messages.*
>
> *Despite losing her hair to chemotherapy and at times having to use a wheelchair, Sophie Foxley writes an account of her day each night and posts it on her site.*
>
> *She tells of how she was first diagnosed with acute lymphoblastic leukaemia on June 8.*
>
> *Sophie, who lives with her parents Phil and Jane, in Bicton Heath, Shrewsbury, details her numerous hospital appointments although her main concern is when her friends can next come round to play as her immune system is often too weak for visitors.*
>
> *As soon as her daughter was diagnosed, Mrs Foxley, 37, gave up her job as deputy manager at the Four Crosses Hotel, Bicton, to look after her full-time.*
>
> *Mrs Foxley said: 'Sophie had not been sleeping very well. She had banged her knee and had a big bruise and pains in her legs.*
>
> *'She was sent straight to the hospital and following a blood test, she was diagnosed with leukaemia.'*
>
> *Sophie's 14-year-old brother Tom came up with the idea for the online blog to help his sister's friends and family keep up to date with her news.*
>
> *Although she has undergone many operations and chemotherapy sessions, she has two more years of treatment ahead of her. Visit www.codebrush.com/sophie to read her diary.*

To Sophie,

> *You will not remember me but I remember you well along with all the other staff who looked after you at Earlyworld nursery.*
>
> *You joined us in Peter Rabbits and soon settled in with your winning smile and cheery nature. You enjoyed painting but most of all you enjoyed to talk!!!*
>
> *You were always keen to tell us about your weekends with Tom and Jenny at circle time and chat to your friends in the quiet corner when you were supposed to be reading (!).*
>
> *If ever an errand needed doing you were always the first child to offer to do it and we could rely on you to carry it out, thank you.*
>
> *You were not with us long before school beckoned and off you went with confidence without so much as a backward glance – at this point our part in your formative education was complete.*
>
> *Those who remember you at Earlyworld were saddened to read about you in the Star today but join me in wishing you well and want you to know that you are in our thoughts.*
>
> *We are going to follow your progress in your online journal (so that is what blogging is all about!). I am sure that you will be an inspiration to anyone who reads about you.*
>
> *Take care,*

From Nicola Crawford and all at Earlyworld XXXXXX

Dear Sophie,

Anyone as brave as you deserves to get better. Wishing you all the very best for the future and hope all goes well for you and your family.
Love and luck,

John and Elaine

Dearest Sophie,

You are such a brave little girl. I hope you get well soon and will follow your story. Good luck to you and your mum and dad. xxxx

Sharnia

Dear Sophie,

We have read about you in the Shropshire Star. Be strong and happy you will make it. Good luck and best wishes.

The Carley family in Holland

Hi Sophie,

Just writing to tell you that five years ago in July 2001 my little boy was diagnosed with ALL [acute lymphoblastic leukaemia] the same as you. He was then only four years old.
He has now had all his treatment and has been off all his medicines for the last two years. He also had all his treatment at Shrewsbury and Birmingham and loved all the doctors and nurses.
He is now nine and doing well off treatment and enjoying life to the full. I wish you all the best for the future and you never know we might see you sometime at clinic.
The Darling family

Dear Sophie and family,

I was just a bit older then your brother and sister when my Dad was told he had cancer, so I know how they feel sometimes.
The best way we have coped with this time is that we have laughed our way though it's been nearly five years now and he's still here.
My Dad has never hid the fact he has cancer and has been proud with it. So when people look a certain way at you, stand up proud.

And for the rest of the family remember, laughter is the best medicine.

All the best and get well.
Luv, Anon

My dearest Sophie,

I have just read your diary and realise what a mature and very brave little girl you are, I'm sure with the help and guidance of all your lovely friends and family and the care of the hospital you will surely make a complete recovery.

> *There must be days when you are a little down but think positively Sophie*
> *and things will get better.*
> Christine xxx

The benefits of the blog flow in both directions: people like Sophie get the opportunity to write about their experiences and the support and encouragement of others, and service designers, if they care to look, get some wonderful insights in to the sick child's world, and rich material for building improvements into their hospitals and surgeries.

Sophie is not unique. There is now a host of specialist children's websites, like *Bandaides*, for example, where you can read Trudy's remarkable story about her 22 operations and daily battle with incontinence ('I also have a pouch on my belly where the urine comes out, and most of the time it's OK, but occasionally it leaks. Now that's a problem, because the kids can smell it sometimes, and they say, "someone blew one"'); or Anthony's story about his leukaemia and how the kids at school called him 'fat cheeks' and 'blow up boy' (www.lehman.cuny.edu/faculty/jfleitas/bandaides). The potential of these stories within the framework of EBD is limitless, we believe.

In Chapter 9 we shall describe our own rather more modest attempts at harnessing the power of the internet for EBD.

Videotaping: 'the storytelling laboratory'

Building on the narrative approach, Dr James Espinosa and colleagues at the US Atlantic Health System have been using video-based storytelling and other narrative medicine strategies in interesting and creative ways to study, design and improve clinical services.[28] One approach involved videotaping patients telling their stories of 'what went well and what didn't go so well', 'what felt safe and what did not feel safe' or 'what satisfied or delighted and what did not', subsequently replaying these stories at hospital quality meetings or back in the departments that had given the treatment (we adopted a very similar approach in the case study – *see* Chapter 9). Another approach was the use of video process map 'walk-throughs': a macro process map was prepared in advance and followed by a video walk through of the process *in vivo*. This was then used as part of a 'safety summit', focusing on problem areas and using frequent 'stop-action' pauses for discussion and dialogue. The result was improved problem-solving and a renewed commitment to safety/quality concerns. Video was also used to produce full-length films about chosen subjects in the quality or safety design field. This involved a number of common steps:

- establish the aim and locus of interest
- construct a storyboard of the story (sketches, flow charts, pictures)
- decide on the cast ('real' people or actors)
- decide locations for shoot
- list the props needed to make the shoot realistic
- identify the production team (amateurs or professionals)
- shoot
- decide on diffusion strategy and outcome measures.

More important than the actual technology was the learning process they put around it, which drew on the Brechtian notions of the 'Theatre for Instruction', in which participants could be enabled by the video to disengage ('alienate'/ *Verfremdung*) themselves from their 'obvious' everyday ways of looking at the world, and to be more reflective, thoughtful and critical of their taken-for-granted world – the notion of learning and developing critical consciousness by observing oneself acting. The parallels with the phenomenology of experience discussed earlier are clear, and it is interesting to see how video can be used in practical ways such as this to get into the difficult area of experience.

One further example – this time going under the name of 'videoethnography' – is a case study of the use of videotaping in a spinal pressure clinic in Australia.[29] This research focused on the impact a redesign of the clinic had on the relationships (a) between the spinal clinicians and (b) with their patients. One aspect of everyday life in the clinic which the video captured were the high number of conversations that went on between clinical staff in corridors. This observation raised important patient (and staff) safety issues:

> *Upon viewing the corridor conversations on the screen, the clinic's infection-control clinician became alerted to the infection risks these conversations pose. Because the clinic deals with wounds and infections, and given the dangerous increase in incidences of multi-resistant organisms, infection control here is crucial. The video data enabled the infection-control clinician to identify previously unrecognised environmental risk factors, such as mobile phones and other equipment handled and exchanged in the corridor and representing potential vectors of infection transmission. This led to the realisation that clinicians' heterogeneous corridor interactions create additional cross-infection risks, due to clinicians moving from patient room to patient room, stopping to talk to each other, and touching and exchanging objects in the corridor. She concludes: 'Whereas when I've observed and been in there, there's so much activity that it's difficult to focus on anything. Seeing the video you can really focus and break things down. It's great. It's much better than doing audits ...'[29]*

As a result of these and other changes that were made, the authors suggest that 'video-based research may provide staff with new resources and opportunities for shaping their increasingly public and visible work practices'.[29]

Focus groups and listening labs

Traditional usability research makes extensive use of focus groups[30] and listening labs, the latter of which may be a group of people or one-on-one, with individuals recounting their experiences, viewed from behind a glass:

> *They are open-ended, qualitative one-to-one sessions that capture both strategic and tactical customer insights. Over the course of one or two days, a typical lab will test a total of six to eight customers in one-on-one sessions that last 45 minutes or longer ... listening labs are designed to emphasize the behaviour and actions of customers, not primarily their opinions ... listening labs do not focus on the highly scripted, task-based methods of traditional usability tests.[31]*

Later this may lead on to active involvement of users in prototyping new designs – (see, for example, www.creativegood.com/casestudies/ae.html, accessed 3 August 2006), although as we have already said it is usually a case of the user being consulted rather than involved as co-designers in the product or service development phase. Hurst's book is useful because it shows how such a situation can be avoided and listening labs made an integral part of a customer experience strategy and process.[31]

For those who are not familiar with focus groups, Rosenbaum gives a useful thumbnail sketch of the essentials:

> *Usability focus groups apply a method that originated in market research to obtain qualitative information from target users. In a focus group, people with similar characteristics who don't know one another meet in a group environment, where they discuss a selected topic with the assistance of a moderator. The goal of the focus group is to have its members interact and spark ideas from one another. Successful focus groups produce a variety of ideas, not a consensus of opinion; the purpose of a focus group is not to make decisions but to collect information. Usability focus groups are task-based and add user tasks and activities to the traditional discussions.*[11]

The web-based focus group is another recent development, which although widely used by private companies today has yet to make an appearance in healthcare or the public sector. One interesting documented example is Intuit, the multinational corporation, which used a web-based focus group to help turn around the fortunes of one of its ailing companies, TurboTax:

> *Intuit turned around TurboTax's online market-share slide by, in part, institutionalizing its ability to constantly improve its offerings. The company's Consumer Tax Group, which had seen the biggest share decline, created a 6,000-member 'Inner Circle' of customers who agreed to serve as a kind of ongoing, Web-based focus group. They supplied basic demographic information, along with their response to the all-important question 'How likely are you to recommend TurboTax to friends or colleagues?' They were then asked to explain their No. 1 priority for enhancing service in any aspect of the customer experience, including shopping, buying, installing, and using tech support. A follow-up question let them prioritize a list of ten suggestions made by other customers.*
>
> *Thanks to these moves, the Consumer Tax Group was able to redesign its core TurboTax product, deliver it to the customer more effectively than ever, and maintain a mechanism for continually developing its related capabilities. Net promoter scores among both first-time users and veterans rose dramatically, and the company regained market share in Web-based channels and renewed share growth in stores.*[32]

Extended focus groups: patients as teachers

Some impressive work has recently been taking place in Lambeth, Southwark and Lewisham Health Authority under the heading of the 'Patients as Teachers' programme (PAT).[33] This has taken focus groups closer toward the co-design end of the spectrum, at the same time building the relationship described earlier where patients have become the teachers and the professionals their students. It is worth recalling the comments we made about the need for such a role reversal in the EBD process in order to allow patient experience to surface:

> *Therefore, in an interesting role reversal, the patient becomes the expert, the instructor or educator, mentor to you the mentee, master to apprentice. No longer are they your 'subject'. They are now the main characters in the play and you are their understudy.*

Being one of the few studies to bring about a partial fusion of EBD and focus groups, the Lewisham work is worth describing in some detail. The chosen design for two experiments with cardiac and later mental healthcare patients was neat, and the method for getting at experience simple but effective. Also, as befits an EBD process, the focus was on positives rather than negatives.

The patients as teachers process involves delegates from patient focus groups meeting professionals to discuss 'what works' from their own point of view. The process has been carried out in cardiac care and mental health.

1   Four focus groups of patients all of whom suffered from IHD [ischaemic heart disease] were recruited from local general practices. One group consisted of women (mixed ages), one of men (under 65), one of older people (mixed gender, over 65 years), and one was a group of people from the Asian community. These groups are known to have differences in clinical presentation and outcomes. The groups were asked: 'In your experience, what has worked best for you in the management of your heart disease?' This approach was designed to elicit constructive comment on the quality of care, based on the individual experiences of the participants. The groups were professionally facilitated, discussions taped, transcribed and summarised.

2   Self-selected delegates were identified. They were now asked not to speak about their personal experiences, but to represent the views of all those in their focus group.

3   The groups then met with primary care clinicians and taught them good practice from the patients' points of view. Professionals, 20 GPs and 6 nurses in two professionally facilitated meetings, were encouraged to listen and be receptive to patients' views. Summaries and recommendations from the focus groups were provided to both users and professionals.

The professional participants were surveyed after 6 months and asked what changes, if any, they had implemented as a result of the meeting.[33]

Fisher subsequently reported, first, on the proportion of recommendations that were put into practice and, second, on the aspects of the 'consultation style' that had changed since the last group meeting.[33] Substantial change in self-reported behaviour was evident, including involvement in treatment decisions (for example, through provision of information), practice management issues (reducing phone interruptions, offering flexible appointment lengths) and continuity of care (referrals to rehabilitation care). All patients (100% response rate) found the meetings interesting and useful. Ten (66%) gained new information from the meetings. None found them frightening or felt there were issues that they could not raise. Eighty per cent of practitioners (90% response rate) found the meeting 'fairly' or 'very' useful, although 43% also said they gained little from the meeting. The authors thus concluded:

Compared to other educational interventions that show little effect on professional change this patient-mediated intervention appears to have had a significant impact on practice.

The difference between this and the, less impactful, DIs method is therefore quite marked, possibly because the Lewisham experiment was much more explicitly focused on redesign and changing practices.

Patient–Professional Action Teams

In what has been described as 'never being a more difficult challenge for experience design'[34] the NHS's £6 billion National Programme for IT (NPfIT) – now Connecting for Health – has set up the Care Record Development Board to jointly represent the interests of clinicians and patients. Going beyond being a mere 'talking shop' it has established core 'action teams' to *define* processes within health and social care that can benefit from IT (information technology). These teams are made up of a broad mix of patient users along with the professionals. While still too early to say (and the language still being very much of the 'consultation and input' kind), these teams have at least the potential to move over time from *define* to *design*. Nevertheless, even the idea of bringing EBD to IT design, development and implementation is an exciting one.

Conversation archives[35]

Electronic communications have opened up new opportunities for gathering ongoing 'persistent conversation' in human-to-human interaction,[36] that is to say the routine, everyday verbal exchanges embodied in email, message texting, electronic reports (e.g. notes of patient examination) and other forms of electronic networking and recorded communication. 'Persistent conversation' is information on e-networks and digital media (personal email, chatrooms, special interest groups (SIGs), multiple user dimensions (MUDs), news groups, web boards, etc.) that leaves a permanent trace (the memory pack for a project), capturing the minutiae of interaction, different viewpoints, and a chronology of events. Analysis of these computer-mediated conversational practices (CMCs – computer mediated communication systems) has opened up new avenues to social scientists and anthropologists, who have previously been confined to written documents and formal and informal face-to-face talk[36] (for example, *see* the papers in the minitrack of the Proceedings of the Hawaii International Conference on Systems Sciences (HICSS), 1999–2004). Once 'copied in', researchers can build a 'conversation archive' around the project.[35] So, whereas in the past most of this everyday material (recalling Heidegger, the very stuff of everyday experience that we are after) would have been lost for ever, it can now be retrieved in the form of a rich 'conversation archive'[35] and replayed at will. A striking example of this was a recent commission undertaken by the authors to research and write up the 'story' of a well-known government agency. A visit to head office revealed the usual ton of documents and minutes, but what we had not expected was the record that had been kept of every email and communication passing between agency members over the past five years. Such an experience brought heightened meaning to (anthropologist) Malinowski's concept of 'living history'!

EBD models, techniques, exercises and interventions

Although the division is not so clear-cut, the methods described above are mostly concerned with helping to diagnose and identify issues for improvement through a better understanding of 'experience' rather than interventions in their own right. We now move on to briefly review some common interventions for improving those experiences, in which we see diagnosis turned into a design process and a sequence of activities that is intended to lead to real change.

The POSE model and other 'step' or 'sequence' models of design

This is an overarching model of EBD that describes the sequence of developmental targets in the EBD process, from initial problem to embodiment or realisation. **P** stands for defining or framing the *problem*; **O** stands for identifying *opportunities*, which brings an understanding of experience together with organisational or departmental goals or objectives; **S** stands for inventing *solutions*; and **E** stands for creating *embodiments*, in which particular solution concepts are designed and given material form.[37]

The design company IDEO uses a four-step design process[38] that is similar to this, which being fairly generic can apply to EBD or any other kind of design process.

- Step one: understand and observe (service and context of use).
- Step two: visualise (sketches, models and prototype solutions).
- Step three: evaluate and refine (detailed prototypes).
- Step four: implement (bench testing and final tooling).

ISO 13407 proposes a similar sequence to this one of 'user centred design activities' that need to start at the earliest stage of the project.[39]

- Step one: understand and specify the context of use.
- Step two: specify the user and organisational requirements.
- Step three: produce design solutions.
- Step four: evaluate designs against requirements.

In an interesting example of ethnography and interaction design working together – and again similar to the above – Brooke and Burrell[3] describe a project to introduce computing methods into a vineyard that was divided into four phases:

- research (the now familiar semi-structured interviews with all the major players and participant observations, including helping with the grape harvest and crush)
- concept development (ideas emerging from the first phase about battery-driven minicomputers and a wireless network to transmit sensing data (weather, ripeness, pests, etc.))
- prototype development (drawings, demos, sketches and mock-ups), and
- assessment (informal feedback to vineyard managers and others).

Most of these EBD 'step' models have been developed and used outside the healthcare field (and would therefore need to be adapted) but there are one or two exceptions, including our wider NHS work, to which we would like to draw readers' attention. In a paper related to the broader debate regarding the design sciences that we mentioned in the Preface to this book, colleagues and ourselves describe how a team of researchers and practitioners have been working together both to explore and to apply 'design sciences' thinking to leading improvement and change in a healthcare context.[40] Using empirical data from the system-level of the NHS as a case study, the paper describes how design sciences can, first, expand thinking around organisational theory and practice, and, second, can possibly offer healthcare some new methods, approaches and processes around the 'doing' of large-scale change. The most relevant part of that work for here – and based on a review of the

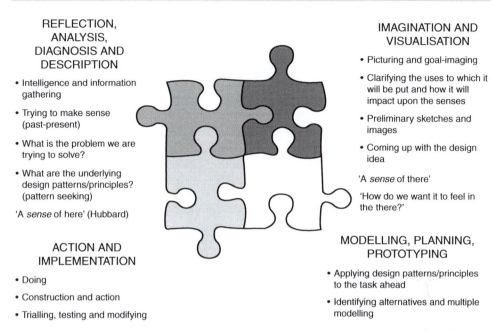

REFLECTION, ANALYSIS, DIAGNOSIS AND DESCRIPTION

- Intelligence and information gathering
- Trying to make sense (past-present)
- What is the problem we are trying to solve?
- What are the underlying design patterns/principles? (pattern seeking)

'A *sense* of here' (Hubbard)

IMAGINATION AND VISUALISATION

- Picturing and goal-imaging
- Clarifying the uses to which it will be put and how it will impact upon the senses
- Preliminary sketches and images
- Coming up with the design idea

'A *sense* of there'

'How do we want it to feel in the there?'

ACTION AND IMPLEMENTATION

- Doing
- Construction and action
- Trialling, testing and modifying

MODELLING, PLANNING, PROTOTYPING

- Applying design patterns/principles to the task ahead
- Identifying alternatives and multiple modelling

Figure 8.1 Thinking like a designer. *Source:* Bevan *et al.*[40]

design literature and an analysis of 'how designers think' – is an intervention model we devised that breaks down the design process into four stages beginning in the top left: reflect, visualise, prototype and then implement (*see* Figure 8.1).

The model is fuller and more detailed than the others described above but still retains the basic 'research–ideas–models–testing–evaluation' structure found in them all and in the design field generally. Clearly, there are also similarities and overlaps with the '*n*-step' models typically found in OD and change management (*see* Collins for a wonderful review and critique of *n*-step guides to change[41]), and especially with the well-known 'action research' model, but we would suggest three main differences:

(a) at stage one, which is retrospective or 'past state' rather than the more usual 'present state' focus of OD

(b) the greater stress in stage two on imagination and creativity than 'vision' or 'plan' and

(c) the special importance attached in design at stage three to building and 'field-testing' prototypes of varying degrees of sophistication (low fidelity to high fidelity).

Of course the biggest difference as far as EBD is concerned is that OD and action research have had little interest in 'experience' up until now, preferring a much more 'etic' and behavourist orientation.

Cognitive walkthrough

This is a review process where scenarios or 'journey maps' (www.ideo.com) are created 'in the mind', with an evaluator playing the role of a typical user, or better still the user him- or herself, 'walking through in the head' and trying to imagine what a new design might feel like, as though the prototype had already been built.[42] One popular focus is upon the things that block progress, that represent emotional and cognitive 'pressure points' for the user. Methods like these can be accompanied by card sorts and storyboards (*see* below).

Card sorts

Card sorting is a method used to get at the cognitive structures or constructs in people's heads: how they categorise, prioritise, and organise. Card sorts are usually conducted in one-to-one sessions using materials such as 3×5 index cards, each labelled with a word or phrase that denotes different aspects of that experience. Participants sort and group them in ways that make the best or most sense to them, thereby revealing their 'construct map' around a service or product.

Storyboards

Storyboards are summary descriptions of the different stages of the process or experience journey, and can vary from cartoons and bubbles to detailed descriptions of each separate stage. The purpose of the storyboard is to concentrate on the order and sequencing of things, and how they link up (or not) to each other.[43] Visualisation methods like this – along with working demonstrations, video-dramatisations and screen-based simulations – are being used increasingly by designers to represent and communicate the more experiential aspects of design.[44] Other things are also beginning to change in this area, the early storyboards relying upon a mainly passive audience whereas the newer methods tend to be much more user-active and interactive, with live video-feeds and simulations that are dynamic and organic rather than static and fixed.

Metaphor Elicitation Techniques (MET)

Many EBD techniques, including card sorts and storyboards, start from the assumption that experiences are often so deeply 'locked away' in people's heads and hearts that they cannot simply be tapped and allowed to flow out at will. Rather, they have to be coaxed out, and gradually given fuller shape and form. Zaltman's ZMET technique[45–47] accepts the limitations of direct, rational approaches to the evocation of experience, preferring to use metaphor to capture thoughts, feelings and experiences as they float around in the ether. In this technique, participants collect pictures that represent their thoughts and feelings on a particular area or topic (i.e. the pictures are a visual metaphor). The model is based on a number of premises: most communication is non-verbal; thoughts occur as images; thoughts, feelings and experiences co-mingle; and our senses provide important metaphors that, with patience, can be re-represented or at least validated in words.

Creating an experience motif or haiku

This technique or procedure may come early on in an EBD process when staff or patients are meeting on their own to reflect on their experiences, or later when they come together to share those reflections and co-design the service.

As Berry and colleagues put it, the method involves the creation of an 'experience motif.'

> The experience motif is ideally a three-word expression of what customers [or staff] desire feeling in an experience. The use of three words as opposed to more words or a sentence is to keep the expression simple and focused so that it can be an effective tool to use in the assessment, design, development, and management of experience clues. Otherwise, the motif may in effect become more like a conventional mission statement making the interpretation considerably less focused and more diffuse. The motif becomes the North Star – the foundation for integrating and reconciling all elements of the experience.[48]

A variant of this, developed by one of the authors, is to ask the group to compose a Japanese *haiku* that encapsulates and expresses the very core of the desired experience ('how it must be/feel?'). The haiku is a traditional form of Japanese poetry, limited to 17 syllables and consisting of three metrical units of five, seven, and five syllables. As with the 'motif' method, the limitation on the number of words allowed in the haiku means that only the bare essentials – literally the core essence – can be included, thereby giving the 'vision' of the perfect experience greater (and sometimes frightening) sharpness and clarity.

Scenario-based development (SBD)

Scenario-based development (SBD) is a promising and widely used technique in interactive system design. Scenarios are mocked-up or imagined narrative descriptions about people and their activities and experiences,[49] prototypes and representations of real life issues and events. This activity can be accompanied by storyboards (*see* above). One of the criticisms of tools like this, and their sister methods such as personas and brainstorming, has been that they tend to be based upon the cognitive or functional elements of what users want or need, or may lead to unvalidated assumptions about users – caricatures, not the real thing.[50] This is why it is important to have the users present and participating in the scenario-building process itself, in other words that SBD and EBD come together.

Creating personas

Personas are simply pretend users of the system you are building. You describe them, in a surprising amount of detail, and then design your system for them (which you can also do the EBD way with a sample of the real users of the system). Each cast of personas has at least one primary persona, the person who must be satisfied with the system or service you deliver. Since you cannot build everything for every persona, the establishment of the primary persona can be critical in focusing the design team's efforts effectively.[51,52] Drawing on first-hand experiences with her design team, Hourihan has described some of the possible benefits of creating personas:

> Any time the word 'user' was mentioned, questions flew: 'What user? Who is she and what's she trying to do?' Our work with personas increased our awareness of our audience and their varying skill levels and goals ... The use of personas helped move all our discussions ... away from the realm of vagaries and into tangible, actionable items.[52]

Whether done formally or informally, persona creation is a device that makes it easier for the designer to think about the service from the user's viewpoint rather than their own, and to challenge their own taken-for-granted assumptions about the way the service is and should be (hence the clever title of Hourihan's article 'Taking the "you" out of user'). Personas are very much the domain of designers and the field of design at the moment, but we believe that this method, possibly more than any other, has a lot to offer to the field of healthcare service improvement.

High- and low-fidelity prototypes

Prototypes are trial design solutions, representations of a design made before final artefacts exist.[51,53] They can be of the rough and ready 'low-fidelity' type, scribbles, sketches, and cardboard cut-outs for example,[54] or 'high-fidelity' cleaned-up schematics, diagrams and working models. As the design process moves through its development life cycle, it tends to be represented by a series of prototypes of increasing fidelity; indeed it is this process of moving from one to another that allows it to creep up on its goal.[55]

Prototypes are important because they establish a tactile (hands-on) relationship with the product or service, literally enabling the user to get a feel for it. Several groups of designers and researchers, notably Apple Computer, Xerox Parc, and Interval Research, have been active in pushing the boundaries of prototypes beyond the range of traditional methods.[56,57] Prototyping rarely happens in isolation but is usually one of a sequence of steps in the overall design process (*see* page 99).

Designers will also talk about 'rapid prototyping' which is kept deliberately messy, ambiguous and incomplete so as to encourage creativity and clarity to emerge. It is also left unresolved for as long as possible so as to keep all the options open:

> *It allows a very low-risk way of quickly exploring multiple directions before committing resources to the best one ... Rapid prototyping gives an organisation license to explore hunches or directions that may in turn give more clarity to the problem statement. It also helps organisations to continue to be mindful of the possibilities of creating systemic solutions.*[12]

Prototyping links to two wider ideas that, say Boland and Collopy,[58] could usefully be transferred from the world of designers to that of managers (including, we believe, improvement managers): the first, the importance of maintaining multiple models of a design object (multiple prototypes); the second, the need to be comfortable with both liquid and crystal states. To some extent prototyping is the method that helps and allows both of these things to happen.

Experience prototyping

The American design organisation IDEO have sought to extend prototyping into the world of experience design, hence the title of the approach: 'experience prototyping' (EP). 'Experience', they tell us (as we know), is a complex multisensory phenomenon. For example, think about the experience of a run down a mountain on a snowboard which depends on the weight and materials of the board, the bindings of your boots, the snow conditions, the weather, the air temperature, your skill level, your current state of mind, your companions, and much more. Prototyping (above) is a simplification, extraction, representation, and approximation of these complex sensations into a broader 'look and feel' of how it was or felt. EP is also this, and may use similar methods such as storyboards and video, but differs in allowing designers and users to experience it themselves, rather than passively witnessing a demonstration or someone else's experience.

> *One of the basic tenets of the concept is that experience is, by its nature, subjective and the best way to understand the experiential qualities of an interaction (between a user and the product or service) is to experience it subjectively.*[53]

The philosophy of EP is 'exploring by doing', the focus being upon sensory impact – the 'essence' of a product or service – rather than objective features. EP is as much an attitude as a set of techniques, and a new way of engaging with design based on 'imagined experience'. It involves three sets of activities.

Understanding existing user experiences

This involves building upon designers' own imaginations and the use of proxy devices to recreate the essential elements of a personal experience that would not otherwise be available. A real healthcare example the authors cite is the design of an internet-enabled cardiac telemetry system, where in order to make this the most positive experience possible for the user, they needed to understand what it was like to be a defibrillating pacemaker patient, or not knowing where and when defibrillating shock will occur. Clearly it was not possible for the design team to experience this directly (!) so they did a mock-up for themselves using pagers that simulated the shock of defibrillation. Other methods (for example, designing a new rail service) might include role playing (different kinds of passengers, for example 'pretend you can't speak English'), 'bodystorming' (physically situated brainstorming – on the train itself), and random scenarios (where a design team member is given an instruction such as 'buy a return ticket for yourself and your child ... now do it with gloves on').

Exploring and evaluating design ideas

The second stage involves the use of crude props to create the experience of a new product or service, for example a smooth pebble, joystick or skateboard to explore what different kinds of physical involvement with a computer game might be; a mock-up of an aircraft cabin that uses (and plays with) ordinary chairs (two, three or four to a row, different gaps and pitches) and beds (head to head, head to toe) to simulate the experience, or model an entirely new experience: 'what would it feel like if ...?' Initially, EP is most likely to be 'low fidelity' but can become high fidelity over time with greater sophistication of diagnosis and design. In a way, this is no different from any other kind of prototyping but what makes EP different is that the focus is not so much on sorting out the logistics or ergonomics, but how the experience is likely to 'feel.'

Communicating ideas

Using 'look-and-feel' prototypes to enable the user to imagine how the new product or service will be experienced.

So far, EP has been used mainly by designers for designers, to help them get into the 'skin' of the patient in order to find out how the service appears and is experienced by them. However, there is no reason why it could not also involve the users themselves to a far greater extent than has hitherto been the case, hence eliminating the need for a stage three.

Heuristic evaluations

Heuristic evaluation[42] is a traditional 'expert evaluation' method that involves having a small number of evaluators examine the interface between service and user, and judge it against recognised usability principles (the 'heuristics'). This tends to be used for external audit, having those highly prized features of being independent, objective, and scientific. Heuristic evaluations by two or more usability specialists can identify a majority of the usability problems of a service or product, with the problem identification percentage increasing as you add evaluators. Two evaluators can identify over 50% of the problems, and three can identify about 60%. The curve flattens after five evaluators; it would take 15 evaluators to identify 90% of usability problems.[11] Although, as the term implies, this method is mainly thought about in the context of programme evaluation (and should therefore be in Chapter 10 not here) it can also be an intervention in itself. EBD, in particular, would find it hard to resist a process that has identified 90% of usability problems, and would undoubtedly want to use the results of an heuristic evaluation formatively to proceed with fixing these problems.

Pseudocode

We have all struggled with car repair and computer manuals and instructions for self-assembly furniture that seem to have been put together so as to be as user-unfriendly as possible. One of the reasons for this is that it perhaps did not occur to the designers of the manuals to think deeply about the user, or try to put themselves in the user's shoes. Services can suffer as much from this as a product or artefact. Thinking back to the design patterns method (Chapter 7), one way to approach the problem is to write the pseudocode your users would want, and then make it work with as few additions as possible.[59] An even better way is to get your users to sit down with you and write the pseudocode for – in our case – the clinical services they are receiving. This does not mean giving users full and free rein – the customer is not always right, says Arnold – but of pooling and synthesising both expert and folk (experience-based) knowledge, and coming up with a service that is first rate in clinical and human terms.

The 'path of expression' approach

A number of the methods and exercises we have discussed come nicely together in a specific EBD approach designed by Gage and Kolari[50] that involves asking users, or users and providers, to imagine the future based upon their needs and aspirations: the path of expression. It is through touch points (more below) that one gains access to the dreams and imaginations of the target users, and because this is done through storytelling it is possible to access people's latent sense of what they want in a way that may not be easily expressed through conversations or interviews. The process involves between four and eight people over one to five days of intensive, fast-paced, exciting and energising activity aimed first at helping users build emotional connections to the product or service experience and then designing solutions that appeal to and match their dreams and imaginations. The props and features of the process are as follows.

- Low-tech tools that resemble items in the elementary school classroom or *Blue Peter* studio! (Scissors, glue, poster boards, index cards, sticky notes, pictures, felt pens, cameras, Lego pieces, etc.) These are used to create models, collages or images of the present and ideal situations.
- Storytelling: people may describe an experience, focusing on how it *felt* at the time, and what would have made it feel better at various touch points.
- Design team (system designers and developers) and users work together to build paper prototypes, scenarios, and mock-ups to simulate possible solutions.

The path of expression therefore looks as shown in Figure 8.2.

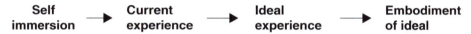

Figure 8.2 The path of expression. *Source*: Gage and Kolari.[50]

The first step is to get the participants immersed in and aware of their daily experiences surrounding the chosen area of focus. A variety of self-expression and documentation exercises can be applied, such as scrapbooks or storytelling exercises in order to bring latent experiences into their conscious memory. In the case of a service consisting of a number of steps this is where one may begin the process of pulling out from the anecdotes and stories and then mapping the various touch points, all of which can be done on flip charts or wall posters (*see* Chapter 9) with pens, post-its, photographs and low-tech tools of various kinds.

In the second step, the participant begins to express his or her feelings to the group and the possible causes through a collage of emotive words and images (another activity that we used to good effect in the EBD case study – *see* Chapter 9). One way to do this is to give each participant an 'emotional honeycomb' sheet showing in each cell a particular one-word emotion (for example, fear, loneliness, hope), positive or negative (previously identified during the interviews), which together provide a mass of emotions from which the participant can make his or her selection and then post these alongside the touch point in question. The emerging map therefore begins to reveal not only the various cognitive experiences associated with the sickness episode but the whole emotional experience rollercoaster that accompanies these.

Asking participants to dream about an ideal or aspired experience is the next step in the process. They may do this by producing another collage that goes alongside the 'present state' one, or may move the pieces around on the present one to model the future 'ideal 'service or product. Very similar to the well-known 'present state/desired state' methods in OD, participants are then able to contrast the two states, and get a sense of the potential for improving the way it could be and feel.

Finally, the process moves on to the designing solutions stage. The intention is that after getting participants to imagine how they want to feel, they are ready to begin to create solutions that will provide their aspired experiences. Such solutions can take the form of simple drawings, maps or prototypes that 'bottle' or embody the essence of that ideal future service or product.

Interestingly, although Gage and Kolari say that 'there is no substitute for the design team hearing and seeing firsthand the ideas generated from the imaginations of the people whom their creativity will ultimately serve',[50] they seem to have forgotten the staff in all this. In their case, being mainly about product design, this may be excusable but in the case of a service where the views and ideas of deliverer and receiver of the service are both crucial, then we believe it is essential to make the design exploratory triadic (patients, staff, designers), a point we return to in the third and final part of this book.

Integrating methodologies for designing the physical environment with those for designing experiences: the story of Manteo

Some readers may be asking themselves where design of the physical environment (say, redesigning the entrance to a hospital or the A&E waiting room) fits in to the overall scheme of an EBD methodology, if anywhere. We take on this issue with a certain degree of reluctance, since 'healing environments' have been covered elsewhere by people with much more expertise in this area than us.[60,61] However, we need to say a few words about how we see EBD and physical design coming together, and describe one particular (as yet largely unused) method that, in our view, goes some way to bridging the gap between the 'physical' objective world and the subjective 'symbolic world' of organisations, blending in very nicely with the overall EBD endeavour.

The reason we need to be doing this at all is the simple fact that physical environment does have a massive impact on all aspects of a design, including (*see* Chapter 1) efficiency and performance (P), safety and reliability (E), and, most importantly here, user experience (A), and it would therefore be impossible, indeed unwise, to ignore it. As we describe in the later case study, by simply redesigning the layout of a clinic or changing the curtains on the ward it is possible to bring about big improvements in patient and user experience. EBD without physical interventions of various kinds is therefore inconceivable, which is why it is important to find a method that simultaneously addresses 'environment' and 'experience', and in a way that recognises this symbiotic, and potentially synergistic, relationship between them.

Sadly, however, a lot of the present physical design work, including healthcare, does not employ anything vaguely approaching an EBD approach. That is to say it neither focuses on patient experience nor provides patient participation in the design of the physical environment. In many, perhaps the majority, of cases today the physical environment is being designed by experts for what they believe the user wants, or is prepared to pay for, not (to recall our earlier phrase) 'with and by' the user – a classic example of 'expert knows best', and a 'designer-centric' approach that flies in the face of EBD, with its user-centric, emic rather than etic, inside-out rather than outside-in, focus. This is why there is a degree of urgency in finding a way to bring physical design and experience design together.

We all have our own examples of what happens when the users, sometimes even staff themselves, are not involved in the design of their immediate physical environment. (Just think of all those disastrous blocks of flats that architects and designers back in the 1950s thought would be great for the residents.) One of our favourite recent examples, a familiar story for many readers, is the NHS trust that established a top-level 'heritage committee', consisting of senior management and board members, architects, designers and professors from an internationally famous college of art to design and commission the artwork and interior and external decoration of its new hospital. Apart from one or two desultory focus groups and exhibitions there was no involvement, directly or indirectly, of users or staff. The sad result of this closed process was a collection of expensive sculptures, paintings, and artefacts that users and staff said they were unable to figure out or understand. More than that, they complained that their space had been invaded by these alien objects. Their experience can best be described as one of bewilderment, and, more seriously for patients encountering the new-age clinic reception desks and areas, confusion and anxiety. Such was the outcry in this particular case that the story reached the national newspapers, which then proceeded to lambast the trust for 'wasting public money'. The only good news to come out of this was that, as a result of this fiasco, the heritage committee was disbanded, the top brass sent away, and the design process brought back in-house. Unfortunately, levels of staff and user participation did not increase significantly as a result, and many of the original artefacts (some now with graffiti additions) remain to this day, as alien to staff and patients as they have always been.

There is clearly a cultural issue here about the elitist mindset that continues to pervade the management and design professions, but we would prefer to concentrate more fruitfully instead on the question of methodology: of how the user's point of view and user experience might be more effectively factored in to the design of the physical environment, so avoiding unfortunate situations like the above from arising. For us the broad challenge can be stated as finding a way of designing the physical environment that is both symbolically and socially meaningful for the actor and recipient, that not only 'makes sense' (and better sense) from their point of view but also actually enhances and improves their immediate experience of that physical situation.

The story of Manteo

Unlikely though this may be as a place to begin, some of the answers, we believe, may be found in the work of landscape architect and University of California professor Randolph T Hester. Hester's work is important because, like EBD, it is an effort to develop community planning that arises from the everyday lives and needs of the insiders of a particular place, not some distant town hall or planner's office (or heritage committee!). The story centres on a particular community design project that Hester carried out during the 1980s for the Outer Banks town of Manteo, North Carolina. The background to the project was a community in crisis. In the 1950s North Carolina had built a bridge to facilitate tourist travel to the beaches of its Outer Banks. While this was a boon to the Outer Banks' tourist trade, it was a slow catastrophe for the town of Manteo, which was bypassed by the new highway and the flow of tourists. Over the next 30 years Manteo changed from the region's principal trade centre to a near ghost town with the highest unemployment and tax rates in the state.

So it was in 1980 that the town of Manteo asked Hester, a community designer, to devise a plan to bring about an economic revival by developing Manteo's historic waterfront to encourage tourism. At the same time, the residents wanted to preserve the aspects of Manteo that they valued; they didn't want to sacrifice the town's character to tourism.

In his ensuing work with the community, which had many of the hallmarks of a rich 'action ethnography' (*see* earlier), Hester discovered that the important places for Manteo residents were not so much its visible, 'formal' buildings, like the church or town hall, but seemingly mundane 'spaces' that were not striking visually or aesthetically, such as a café or tree-lined street. Through the use of behaviour mapping, surveys, and interviews, Hester and his team eventually identified what came to be known as Manteo's 'Sacred Structure' (a name one of the residents, not a designer, came up with) – a set of settings, situations, and events that marked the heart of Manteo as a place for its residents.

'Sacred places'

According to Hester, 'sacred places' are buildings, outdoor spaces, and landscapes that exemplify, typify, reinforce, and perhaps even extol everyday life patterns and special rituals of community life; places that are so essential to residents' lives through use or symbolism that the community collectively identifies them. Their loss reorders or destroys something or some social process familiar to the community's collective being.[62] This Sacred Structure was then used as the basis for Manteo's community design. Later, drawing on this and similar projects, Hester wrote a general primer for community design which, we believe, contains many useful tips for organisation designers today.[63,64]

Later, Hester was to return to Manteo to overview the design process that led to the plan and determine its various successes and failures in the five years since it was implemented.[65] He found that the master design had helped strengthen Manteo's small-town quality, while also strengthening the local economy. He also traced the politics of the town design and found that some residents' opposition to the design had slowed and changed its development. He concluded that, as a design tool, the Sacred Structure provides one way to reduce differences between insiders and outsiders. The importance of Hester's work is that it was able to illustrate one way in which the environmental designer can become a midwife who helps insiders articulate local needs and then translates those needs into design incorporating wider contextual concerns.

Now instead of 'community' think 'organisation', the point being that organisations also have their sacred places, and like Manteo's, these, not the formal structures, should be the focus of design, especially EBD, since the sacred structures to which Hester is referring are not only physical entities, but social, spiritual and aesthetic entities as well. The fact that there is also a cultural dimension to them, in terms of the shared collective sentiments that surround them (they in turn reinforcing these sentiments) also raises the intriguing possibility that EBD interventions directed at 'sacred places' might also be seen as cultural interventions, and might therefore hold some of those elusive keys to cultural change in healthcare. On this point, we hope to be able to show in the case study in Chapter 9 that EBD is not only about improving services, or even experiences, but building culture and community among and between patients, users and staff that sustains them in their life together. Furthermore, it will not have escaped readers' attention that in the Manteo case resistance to change also lessened, a point of some significance as regards staff, especially clinician, engagement and co-operation in healthcare improvement. And finally, going all the way back to our P + E + A model of great design, it seems that Hester's community design model was successful in improving the local economy (equivalent to our P) and the safety of residents (E, re-routing the highway), as well as the quality of the residents' lives (A).

The community design approach

The following gives a little more detail on the two aspects of this community design approach: first, the diagnosis and then the intervention itself. The diagnostic phase begins by asking the 'residents' (obviously, in our case, read staff and patients) what they valued about their community (organisation, department, service). (Readers please note the similarities to Positive Organisational Scholarship and Appreciative Inquiry described earlier.) Initially, Hester used surveys and face-to-face interviews to explore what was important to the residents. These techniques resulted in a number of general findings: people valued small-town qualities such as friendliness and informality; they also saw certain areas (for example, the waterfront) and places (particular shops) as important to their quality of life. So, readers might wish to reflect, if staff and patients were asked what they valued most about their service, what are the kind of things they would say? Our view is that they would not be that dissimilar from the kind of qualities to which the Manteo residents referred – friendliness, informality and so on.

In the event, Hester and his team were not satisfied by these findings. It was not obvious how to move from the general sentiments expressed to decisions about what might be changed and what ought to be preserved. Tom Erickson[66] – currently a researcher and computer interaction designer at IBM who deserves all the credit for reviving Hester's work – takes up the story of what happened next:

> So Hester and his colleagues turned to an approach they called 'behaviour mapping.' This involved observing and recording the activities of the townsfolk over a period of several weeks. The result was a set of sketches of settings and maps of place-based activity that seemed important to the life of community. Mapped behaviours included activities such as 'hanging out at the docks', 'watching the sunset', and 'debating politics in the Dutchess restaurant.' As Hester said, 'Lifestyle and landscape were intertwined. Daily ritual was place-specific, and the cultural dependence on places seemed more widespread than people had reported in our interviews.' It is interesting to note that most of the places in which seemingly important activities were observed had not been mentioned in the surveys or interviews.

This phase is almost identical to the participant observation described earlier in this chapter (page 88), where we referred to 'directly observing people in their natural work habitat, not only talking to them but simply watching them, the value of this in being able to see how they go about their everyday business in real time'. Readers may also have noticed the close similarities between the 'sacred places' concept and the 'touch points' concept; in fact we would go so far as to suggest that sacred places may be defined as touch points with a physical location. More on this later, but let us continue with the story.

The next step was to verify that the places where the activities occurred were actually important to the residents. Using information from the surveys, interviews and behaviour mapping, and drawing on knowledge of social patterns in other towns and discussions with Manteo's leaders, Hester and his team generated a list of 'important places'. The list, in conjunction with a newspaper-based questionnaire, was used to allow the residents to rank the places in order of their importance. The idea was that items above a certain point would be protected from development. The results were collated, and the resulting list was published in the town newspaper. One resident, observing that quite a few places were ranked higher than the local churches and cemetery, dubbed the list 'the Sacred Structure of Manteo'. The name stuck, and came to be used for the places that were to be preserved and protected.

Manteo's sacred structure – eventually codified in a map (*see* Figure 8.3) – consisted of rather mundane places. As Hester notes, 'these places are almost universally unappealing to the trained professional eyes of an architect, historian,

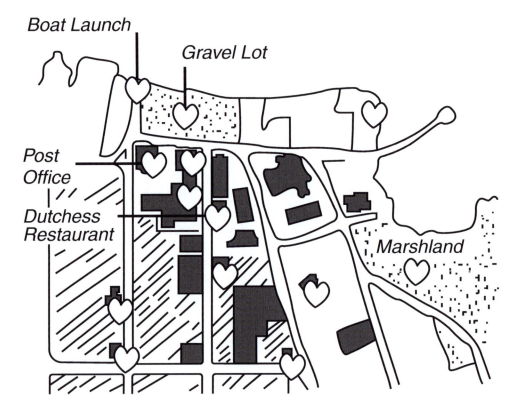

LEGEND

♡ **Sacred Places**

▨ **Sacred Neighborhood**

▦ **Sacred Open Space**

Figure 8.3 Sacred places. *Source:* Erickson.[66]

real estate developer, or upper-middle-class tourist'. For example, the sacred structure included the marshes surrounding the town, a park, the Dutchess restaurant, locally made (unreadable) street signs, and a gravel parking lot where people gathered to watch the sun set and where the town's Christmas tree was set up. Of the sacred places, only two were protected by historic preservation legislation, and a few more by zoning laws; that is, the existing planning and legal mechanisms that were intended to help preserve the character of places missed most of what the residents of Manteo actually valued.

This phrase 'missed most of what the residents of Manteo actually valued' painfully recalls the hospital design fiasco described earlier, but also offers the reminder that the whole point of EBD, with its identical focus on how the 'residents' see it, is to avoid this happening, whether it be in the design of a process, system, or physical space. Our view is that the EBD approach and Hester's could therefore transform the way we currently go about designing the physical settings of healthcare. That being said there are some wonderful exceptions that we have described elsewhere[67] from which there is much to learn, perhaps the most remarkable being the new 140-bed Evelina Children's Hospital at Guy's and St Thomas' in London which has been credited as having been 'created by children for children'.[68] The hospital's very EBD/Manteo-like approach has resulted in a building that, as a design, scores highly on P, E, and A, most notably the latter which, as a result of direct involvement in the design by the young children and their families, has achieved their dream of creating 'a hospital that does not feel like a hospital'.

The Manteo intervention itself is also interesting. As would be expected – and again similar to the Evelina story – this involved lots of participation and lots of talk as the designers mixed and interacted with residents. There were town meetings and public meetings, formal and informal, small and large, but always open and inclusive. 'Sacred places' provided the planning tool, and were used to identify (and prioritise) places that people felt should be left untouched or protected from any new developments, and ruined or run-down outdoor spaces that the community would like to celebrate or do more with (the so-called 'sacked spaces'). For example, a favourite park might become an outdoor theatre, a place for 'learning walks' or the site of a yearly festival, and a drab shopping centre made more attractive through the addition of decorative benches and plantings where employees and shoppers could eat their lunch or simply rest after a long day.

The list of the strengths and achievements of this method is long and impressive:

- It linked physical places to social behaviour and experience, and physical design to social and experience design.
- It got people to engage and participate, and helped overcome indifference and resistance to change.
- It empowered ordinary people because it gave them a language and a method to be able to engage on a level playing field with the designers and the officials, and ultimately to 'do' the designing for themselves. Erickson captures this point perfectly when he describes the sacred places method as a 'lingua franca that is accessible to all, particularly those who are traditionally marginalised in the design process: the users'.[66]
- It provided a way of translating general sentiments into detailed actions.

- It resulted in a design that satisfied the needs and desires of residents and users, and embodied the kind of things they most valued in life.
- It revitalised the community, strengthening its sense of identity and helping bring about widespread and lasting cultural change.
- The (re)development continued even after the designers had left, proof that it had acquired its own energy and momentum, and had given ordinary people the knowledge, ability and motivation to continue.
- Sustainability: the results lasted; when Hester returned five years later he found that the sacred places, and the character of the town generally, had remained intact, and the sacked places eliminated.

Manteo is both a case study and an allegory for EBD, a reminder of what can be achieved when physical design and social design are brought into alignment, and when the needs and experiences of the inhabitants and users themselves are given primacy over all else. It also points to the heart of the EBD challenge, which is how to get a hugely diverse group of stakeholders, staff, patients, designers (and all the varieties within each of these) communicating meaningfully with each other – creating what Erickson calls a linguistic common ground.[66] We now move on to describe how we took up this challenge in a healthcare context, and, with Manteo as our benchmark, how well we fared at the level of practice.

References

1 Fulton Suri J. The experience evolution: developments in design practice. *The Design Journal*. 2003; **6**(2): 39–48.
2 Bell G, Salvador T, Anderson K. Design ethnography. *Design Management Journal*. 1999; **10**(4): 35–41.
3 Brooke T, Burrell J. From ethnography to design in a vineyard. Proceedings of the 2003 Conference on Designing for User Experiences; 2003 June 6–7; San Francisco, California.
4 Anschuetz L, Rosenbaum S. Ethnographic interviews guide design of web site for vehicle buyers. Proceedings of CHI 2003; 2003 April; Fort Lauderdale, FL, USA.
5 Muller MJ. *Participatory Design: The Third Space in HCI, The Human-Computer Interaction Handbook: Fundamentals, Evolving Technologies and Emerging Applications*. Mahwah, NJ: Lawrence Erlbaum Associates; 2002.
6 Millen DR. Rapid ethnography: time deepening strategies for HCI field research. Conference proceedings on Designing Interactive Systems: Processes, Practices, Methods, and Techniques; 2000 August.
7 Beyer H, Holtzblatt K. *Contextual Design: Defining Customer-Centred Systems*. San Francisco, CA: Morgan Kauffman; 1998.
8 Holtzblatt K, Jones S. Contextual inquiry: a participatory technique for system design. In: Schuler D, Namioka A, editors. *Participatory Design Principles and Practices*. Hillsdale, NJ: Erlbaum; 1993. p. 177–210.
9 Kantner L, Hinderer Sova D, Rosenbaum S. Alternative methods for field usability research. *SIGDOC 2003 Proceedings*. San Francisco, CA: ACM Press; 2003.
10 Raven ME, Flanders A. Using contextual inquiry to learn about your audience. *ACM SIGDOC Journal of Computer Documentation*. 1996; **20**(1).
11 Rosenbaum S. Not just a hammer: when and how to employ multiple methods in usability programs. Paper delivered at UPA 2000, sponsored by the Usability Professionals' Association; 2000: 1–2.
12 Coughlan P, Prokopoff H. Managing change, by design. In: Boland RJ, Collopy F, editors. *Managing as Designing*. Stanford, CA: Stanford Business Books; 2004. p. 189.

13 Wood L. The ethnographic interview in user-centred work/task analysis. In: Wixon D, Ramey J, editors. *Field Methods Casebook for Software Design*. New York, NY: Wiley; 1996.

14 Kvale S. *Interviews: An Introduction to Qualitative Research Interviewing*. Thousand Oaks, CA: Sage; 1996.

15 Van Maanen J. Different strokes: qualitative research in the Administrative Science Quarterly from 1956 to 1996. In: Van Maanen J, editor. *Qualitative Studies of Organisations*. Thousand Oaks, CA; Sage; 1998. p. 9.

16 Heyl B. Ethnographic interviewing. In: Atkinson P, Coffey A, Delamont S *et al.*, editors. *Handbook of Ethnography*. London: Sage; 2001.

17 Matrix Consultancy. *Coronary Heart Disease Collaborative. Evaluations of Discovery Interviews: Final Report*. London: Matrix; 2005. p.

18 CHD Collaborative. *Learning From Patient and Carer Experience: A Guide to Using Discovery Interviews to Improve Care*. Leicester: NHS Modernisation Agency; 2004.

19 Jaasko V, Mattelmaki T. Observing and probing. Proceedings of the 2003 International Conference on Designing Pleasurable Products and Interfaces; 2003 June; Pittsburgh, PA, USA.

20 Kuniavsky M. User experience and HCI. Draft chapter at: www.orangecone.com/archives/2006/01/defining_the_us_1.html (accessed 7 September 2006).

21 Denzin NK. *The Research Act*. 3rd ed. Englewood Cliffs, NJ: Prentice Hall; 1989.

22 Flick U. *An Introduction to Qualitative Research*. Sage; London; 1998.

23 McDonald S. Studying actions in context: a qualitative shadowing method for organisational research. *Qualitative Research*. 2005; **5**(4): 455–73.

24 Van Maanen J. *Tales of the Field: On Writing Ethnography*. Chicago, IL: University of Chicago Press; 1988.

25 Erickson T. Design as storytelling. *Interactions*. 1996; **3**(4): 30–5.

26 Hurwitz B, Greenhalgh T, Skultans V, editors. *Narrative Research in Health and Illness*. London: BMJ Publications; 2004.

27 *See* www.shropshirestar.co.uk/2006/08/brave-sophies-story-goes-online/ (accessed 7 September 2006).

28 Maund T, Espinosa JA, Kosnik LK *et al.* Video-storytelling: a step-by-step guide. *Joint Commission Journal on Quality and Safety*. 2003; **29**(3): 152–5.

29 Iedema R, Long D, Forsyth R. Visiblising clinical work: video ethnography in the contemporary hospital. *Health Sociology Review*. 2006; **15**: 156–68.

30 Krueger RA. *Focus Groups: A Practical Guide for Applied Research*. Newbury Park, CA: Sage; 1988.

31 Hurst M. *Joining Strategy and Usability: The Customer Experience Methodology*. New York: Creative Good, Inc; 2003.

32 Allen A, Reichfield FF, Hamilton B. The three 'D's of customer experience. *Harvard Management Update*. 2005; 7 November.

33 Fisher B. *Patients as Teachers – 'What Works For You?' A New Way of Involving Users in Improving Services*. Unpublished paper on two 'patients as teachers' initiatives in Lambeth, Southwark and Lewisham Health Authority. 2005.

34 *See* www.headshift.com/archives/001858.cfm (accessed 3 August 2006).

35 Halverson CA. The value of persistence: a study of the creation, ordering and use of conversation archives by a knowledge worker. Proceedings of the 37th Hawaii International Conference on Systems Sciences; 2004.

36 Erickson T, Herring S. Persistent conversation: a dialog between research and design. Proceedings of the 37th Hawaii International Conference on Systems Sciences; 2004. Also *see*: Persistent conversation. Special issue of *Journal of Computer Mediated Communication*. 1999; **4**(4).

37 Cain J. Experience-based design: towards a science of artful business innovation. *Design Management Journal*. 1998; Fall: 10–14.

38 Bray DD. Creative collaboration: user-centred design in practice. *Medical Device and Diagnostic Industry*. 2000; March: 76–89.

39 *See* www.usabilitynet.org/tools/13407stds.htm (accessed 3 August 2006).

40 Bevan H, Robert G, Bate SP *et al.* Using a design approach to assist large-scale organisational change: 'Ten high impact changes' to improve the National Health Service in England. *Journal of Applied Behavioral Science.* 2007; **43**(1): 135–52.

41 Collins D. *Organisational Change: Sociological Perspectives.* London: Routledge; 1998.

42 Newman WM, Lamming MG. *Interactive System Design.* Reading, MA: Addison-Wesley; 1995.

43 Vertelney L, Curtis G. *Storyboards and Sketch Prototypes for Rapid Interface Visualisation. CHI Tutorial.* New York: ACM Press; 1990.

44 Buur J, Jensen MV, Djajadiningrat T. Hands-on scenarios and video action walls: novel methods for tangible user interaction. Proceedings of the 2004 Conference on Designing Interactive Systems: Processes, Practices, Methods and Techniques; 2004 August; Cambridge, MA: ACM Press. p. 185–92.

45 Zaltman G. Metaphorically speaking. *Marketing Research.* 1996; **8**(2): 13–20.

46 Zaltman G. *How Customers Think: Essential Insights into the Minds of the Market.* Boston, MA: Harvard Business School Press; 2003.

47 Zaltman G, Coulter RH. Seeing the voice of the customer: metaphor-based advertising research. *Journal of Advertising Research.* 1995; **35**(4): 35–51.

48 Berry LL, Wall EA, Carbone LP. Service clues and customer assessment of the service experience: lessons from marketing. *Academy of Management Perspectives.* 2006; **20**(2): 43–57.

49 Carroll J. *Usability Engineering: Scenario-Based Development of Human-Computer Interaction.* San Francisco, CA: Morgan Kaufmann; 2001.

50 Gage M, Kolari P. Making emotional connections through participatory design. *Boxes and Arrows.* 2002; 3 November. Also available on: www.boxesandarrows.com/view/making_emotional_connections_through_participatory_design (accessed 7 December 2006).

51 Cooper A. *The Inmates Are Running the Asylum: Why High-Tech Products Drive Us Crazy and How to Restore the Sanity.* Indianapolis, IN: Sams Publishing; 2004.

52 Hourihan M. Taking the 'you' out of user: my experience using personas. *Boxes and Arrows.* 2002; 26 March. www.boxesandarrows.com/taking_the_you_out_of_user_my_experience_using_personas (accessed 7 December 2006).

53 Buchenau M, Suri JF. Experience prototyping. *ACM.* 2000; 1–58113–219–0/00/0008.

54 Wong YY. Rough and ready prototypes: lessons from graphic design. Proceedings of CHI Posters and Short Talks; 2002 May; New York: ACM Press. p. 79–84.

55 Rudd J, Stern K, Isensee S. Low vs high fidelity prototyping debate. *Interactions.* 1996; **3**(1): 76–85.

56 Burns C, Dishman E, Johnson B *et al.* Informance: minding future contexts for scenario-based interaction design. Presented at BayCHI; 2005 August; Palo Alto. www.baychi.org/meetings/archive/0895.html (accessed 7 September 2006).

57 Burns C, Dishman E, Verplank B *et al.* Actors, hair-dos and videotape: informance design. Presented at Royal College of Art, London; 1997, November.

58 Boland RJ, Collopy F. *Managing as Designing. Bringing the Art of Design to the Practice of Management.* (DVD film.) Information Design Studio, Weatherhead School of Management, Case Western Reserve University; 2004.

59 Arnold K. Programmers are people, too. *Security.* 2005; **3**(5). www.acmqueue.com/modules.php?name=Content&pa=printer_friendly&pid=3 (accessed 30 August 2005).

60 Toren B, Horvath L. Mapping sacred places. Third National Community Impact Assessment Conference. *See* www.trb.org/publications/circulars/ec054/CircEC054%20CIA.pdf (accessed 26 August 2006).

61 Berry LL, Parker D, Coile RC *et al.* The business case for better buildings. *Frontiers of Health Services Management.* 2004; **21**(1): 3–24.

62 Ulrich R. Effects of healthcare interior design on wellness: theory and recent scientific research. In: Marberry S, editor. *Innovations in Healthcare Design.* New York: Van Nostrand Reinhold; 1995. p. 88–104.

63 Hester R. *Community Design Primer*. Mendocino, CA: Ridge Times Press; 1990.

64 Hester R. Wanted: local participation with a view. In: Nasar JL, Brown BB, editors. *Public and Private Places*. Edmond, OK: Environmental Design Research Association; 1996. p. 42–52.

65 Hester RT. Sacred Structures and everyday life: a return to Manteo, NC. In: Seamon D, editor. *Dwelling, Seeing, and Designing: Toward A Phenomenological Ecology*. New York: SUNY Press; 1993.

66 Erickson T. Lingua francas for design: sacred places and pattern languages. In: Boyarski D, Kellogg WA, editors. *Proceedings of the ACM Conference on Designing Interactive Systems*. New York: ACM Press; 2000. p. 357–68.

67 Bate SP, Robert G. Experience-based design: from redesigning the system around the patient to co-designing services with the patient. *Quality and Safety in Health Care*. 2006; **15**(5): 307–10.

68 *See* www.guysandstthomas.nhs.uk/news/newsarchive/newsarticles/echpeopleschoice. aspx (accessed 7 December 2006).

Appendix

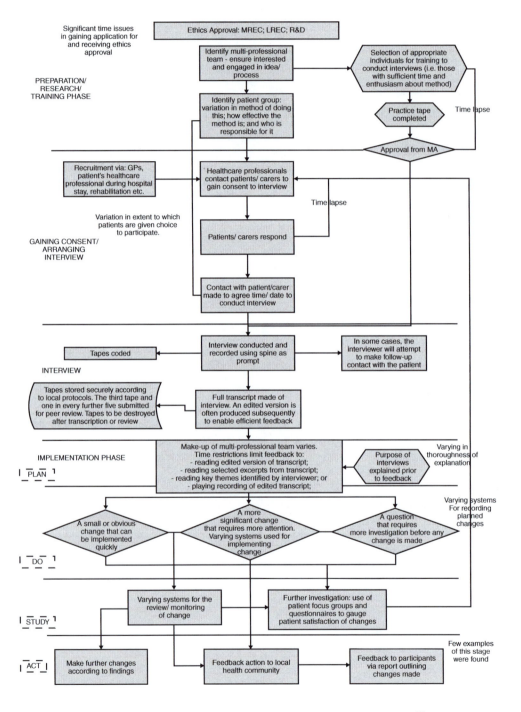

Figure A The Discovery Interview Method. *Source:* Matrix Consultancy.[18]

Part 3

Practices

The third and final part of this book (Chapters 9–10) sees us moving on from discussions of the conceptual (Part 1) and methodological (Part 2) challenges of understanding and capturing 'experience' to the practical challenges surrounding the implementation of an EBD process in a healthcare organisation.

In Chapter 9 we begin with a detailed description of the EBD process as applied in a real-life case study. We examine the 'what' and the 'how' of 'experience mapping' (as opposed to traditional 'process mapping'), at the core of which lies the concept of touch points. The chapter discusses this notion of touch points by means of several examples of these 'moments of truth' based on direct quotations from patients and staff. We then illustrate how patients and staff, working together, can move on to formulate design principles (as discussed in Chapter 7) from these touch points for improving their experiences of a service and embedding the change. The part ends by discussing the importance of evaluating the changes in experience brought about by an EBD intervention (Chapter 10), including reflections on the learning prospectively captured while undertaking the case study and suggestions for how it might be done better next time.

Chapter 9

The 'how' of experience-based co-design: a case study for practitioners

Interviewer: If you were to give us a lead as to where we might begin to improve the patient experience, around Head and Neck cancer, not just the Outpatient Clinic, where would you direct us towards? Where do you think are some of the areas where we could, between us, improve the patient experience?

Consultant surgeon: God, you could write a book about that!

Interviewer: We probably will . . .

The case study

This case study of implementing an EBD approach draws on pilot work undertaken over an intensive 12-month period with head and neck cancer patients, carers and staff to improve services centred around one acute hospital in the south of England. This work combined a number of the diagnostic and intervention methods described in Chapter 8 into a single process and intervention.

Locally the hospital had already had some experience of involving patients in service improvement and of listening to and capturing what they say. There was also a well-established patient-led support group for laryngectomy patients (although no such groups existed for non-laryngectomy patients or head and neck cancer patients generally). This is significant as the presence of patient- (or professionally) led support groups for people with cancer has been identified as important to patient experience (that is, as long as the group provides a supportive environment, mutuality and a sense of belonging and meets other perceived needs).[1]

In the past, different groups of patients had also attended stakeholder events, participated in discovery interviews, completed surveys and mapped healthcare processes with improvement specialists from the hospital. The same staff had visited community groups and spoken to patients and their carers about services and asked them about what would constitute ideal care from their perspective. However, up to that point the work had not really focused on the patient experience beyond asking what was good and what was not. Questions had not been asked that sought to find out what the experience was like and then to use the information systematically to design services *with* patients. The justification for the work was therefore that knowledge of the experience held only by the patient is valuable and unique and analysis of the data would reveal a number of touch points: points during the experience that made or could have made a difference to the experience.

The model of EBD piloted with the head and neck cancer service involved gathering experience-related data from patients and staff (from in-depth interviewing, observation, photography and film), verifying that data with them, identifying the key touch points, using the touch points to describe design principles, and discussing those principles with a group that included the same

patients and staff to design services, and finally moving jointly towards implementation and practical action. As a pilot, the main research question was:

> *Can experience-based design be applied to healthcare processes and practice,*
> *and does this innovative approach improve services and patient experiences?*

The case study was deliberately designed (and funded) as a prototype for testing the value of an EBD approach and was consequently of a longer duration (and
more resource intensive) than we imagine would be possible in a typical hospital.
Further ongoing EBD work in other hospitals is therefore using a scaled-down
model (of six to eight months' duration) based on the lessons learned in the pilot.

In describing the case study in full here, we seek to illustrate how an improvement specialist or OD practitioner might design, utilise and participate in an EBD
approach. Given that the approach itself retains the traditional core of OD (i.e.
EBD can be overlaid on top of a traditional OD intervention) this is not some
great leap forward but rather a reconceptualisation of the OD process and aims.[2]
Our proposition is that it is within the co-analysis and co-design by staff and users
(employing concepts such as 'touch points' and 'design principles') that EBD can
help forge new directions for OD, while at the same time OD can bring change
models and skills to EBD and the design field generally that designers in other
fields may lack.

The EBD process

Figure 9.1 shows the process as employed in the case study and highlights that this
is indeed a co-design process, with both staff and patients involved from the very
outset, first on their own and then together in a close working partnership. Thus,
while EBD is highly 'patient-*centred*' (in aiming to 'make it a better experience' for
patients), it is not patient-*led* as such. Rather, leadership is shared between staff and
patients in what is effectively a process of co-determination based upon a set of
common aims and purposes (the German concept of *mitbestimmung*). Thus, the
innocent little 'co' in co-design puts a big question mark over today's in-phrase
within healthcare – the politically correct but organisationally naive, as well as
imprecise, 'patient-led' – and suggests more of a partnership between patients, carers and staff in the design of services, and not something where staff and staff interests are apparently so marginal and unimportant as not even to receive a mention
in this phrase. The various elements shown in Figure 9.1 are described below.

Core group

In this particular case, the core management or project group consisted of the OD
researchers and evaluators (two in this particular case study), designers (a
graphic designer and a film-maker), internal hospital improvement specialists
(two) and the national sponsor of the project (one). One of the first tasks of the
core group was to formulate a brief description of the project setting out its aim
and purpose:

> *The primary purpose of the research is to test out a model of experience-based*
> *design (EBD). This involves using patients' direct experiences of our services to*
> *design and improve those services. 'Experience' is an extremely valuable source*
> *of knowledge, through which we are able to identify those parts of the treatment*

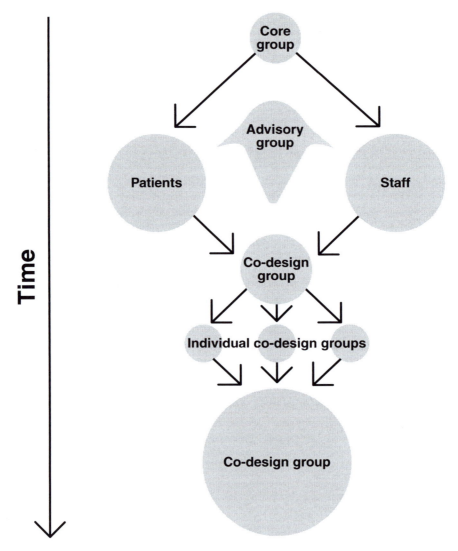

Figure 9.1   The experience-based co-design process.

journey where the patients' feelings of the service – positive and negative – are being most strongly formed ('touch points'), and therefore where improvement efforts need to be focused. Examination of these touch points will enable the team of staff and patients to identify design principles which will then be applied to the redesign and improvement of services for future patients with head and neck cancer.

Advisory group

This group was made up of patient and carer volunteers (four) who were using the service at the time of the case study or had used it in the recent past, plus internal hospital staff: the chief nurse, a general manager, a head and neck (H & N) cancer surgeon and an H & N clinical nurse specialist. The role of the steering group was broadly to 'advise, encourage and warn', and to provide a perform-ance management role in respect of the core group. In practice, however, given that this was an experiment in which everyone was feeling their way, the advi-sory group ended up playing a wider role in helping to agree both the specifics of the EBD approach and the intervention itself. In particular, the chief nurse and medical director played a key role towards the end of the EBD process in align-ing the quality and service improvements identified by patients and staff as pri-orities with the organisation's internal management and performance monitoring systems (*see* 'Reflections', Box E, page 157).

Staff

The EBD process began in typical ethnographic fashion (*see* Chapter 8) with a combination of contextual inquiry, direct observation of the H & N clinic ('organ-isational loitering', *see* page 88) and one-to-one interviews with staff, led by the two organisation researchers but involving other members of the core group in rotation to allow for the transfer of learning to the organisation. The purpose was to enable the core group to hear and learn about the service (think of this also in terms of an induction and familiarisation), the staff's own experiences of it, and how they felt patients also experienced that service. Importantly, this first phase, as we soon discovered, also has a social and professional aim of making contact and building relationships with a sample of key clinical staff to gain support for the project and their commitment to further improve services.

The direct observation included the researchers 'sitting in' on three of the fort-nightly outpatient H & N clinics as well as the multidisciplinary team meetings directly preceding the clinics. The clinics would usually run for four hours during the morning and, typically, one of the researchers would remain in the waiting area observing the general 'comings and goings' of the clinic while the other would shadow (*see* Chapter 8) a key member of the clinic staff including on one occasion the clinical nurse specialist and on another a consultant surgeon. One of the aims of the observations was to capture the minutiae of the various interac-tions and all the mundane 'babble and chat'[3] of everyday conversation between patients and staff; Bradner and colleagues[4] refer to this task as 'constructing an ecology of communicative practices'. In this case study, this observation also included sitting in on approximately 50 'one-to-one' patient/doctor consultations (although as we discuss later such 'one-to-one' consultations are anything but that). Both researchers would take detailed notes of what they saw and heard dur-ing the clinic. Immediately after the clinic the researchers would meet and, on the basis of their notes, dictate an audio diary of what they had observed that morn-ing, as well as ask each other questions in order to identify key observations and emerging issues. These diaries, which were very colloquial and natural, would then be transcribed. The following extract from one of those diaries describing a single patient consultation illustrates the type of data collected during our initial fieldwork using this audio diary method. For readers unfamiliar with the acronym PEG used in this extract, percutaneous endoscopic gastrostomy (PEG) is a proce-dure to insert a feeding tube into the stomach without the need for an operation; the tube allows liquid feeds to be put directly into the stomach.

> *Audio diary: Researcher 1, November 2005. He [Patient 2] came in and he looked dreadful. He'd had diarrhoea for 11 days. His breathing was dreadful.*

He could barely breathe. The last time he was here he didn't want much information. As [the clinical nurse specialist] says, 'I've asked all the questions', and she's annoyed with him because he didn't come sooner. So, she saw all this going on. He wouldn't come sooner. He hates hospitals, he hates the illness, he's a very unhappy man. He's had an MRI but not a PEG. The PEG is next week. He's got to come in for that. He's got oedema – swelling of the neck – but it's mainly because of the tumour that he's got a problem breathing. His wife said he hated the MRI and he's not been the same since and she said, 'He wasn't given enough information about what that experience with the MRI is like. You feel all claustrophobic. Or if you hate the noise, the noise is boom, boom, boom, boom.' And this guy had not been the same since. So, he didn't get information about that other stuff. Then they agreed that this airway that he's got, quote, 'could go any time: you should be admitted'. So, they're looking at this guy and he was really distressed. He doesn't want to. He wants to go back to feed his birds on the lawn. He just doesn't want to know. He hates it. And he's the car driver. His wife doesn't drive. So, 'If I'm admitted now, how are you going to get back?' 'Well, I'll take a taxi' . . . and he's thinking, and, above all, 'I don't want to be admitted now. I only came here for a consultation. I'm coming in in three days time and now you're saying you want to admit me . . .'

In the end [the female H & N surgeon] lets him talk about it and then [the female H & N surgeon] says, 'Well, we need a mobile number for you and we'll get [the clinical nurse specialist] to ring you at home tomorrow to check you're okay.' So, they agreed that and the patient and his wife leave, and then in comes [the clinical oncologist] and she says, 'Have you laid it on the line for him about the dangers of going home now?' And then [the male plastic surgeon] comes in with [the oncologist]. So, there's [the clinical nurse specialist, the oncologist, the H & N surgeon and the plastic surgeon] and they said, 'This guy's got to come in to the hospital because if his airway goes, he's had it basically.' So, in the end they get the patient back in to the room and [the plastic surgeon] then said, '[Patient 2], do you know the risks, if it closes up . . .?', man to man, and straight away, within a second, he says, 'If you say so, doctor', and the doctor says, 'Good man'. So here's the female H & N surgeon trying to give the patient the same advice that [the male plastic surgeon] gives him and he complies straight away with [the male plastic surgeon] but he wouldn't agree with [the female H & N surgeon] . . . So, there is a question in here for me about choice, again. In the end [the female H & N surgeon] gave him the choice of whether to come in or go home. I don't think [the male plastic surgeon] really gave him any choice. There was no choice. Has the patient got the right to say, 'I'm sorry, I'm going to take the risk, the risk is mine, and if I do lose the airway . . .'?

Such observational data – and this is just one extract from hours of our audio diaries – provided early insights into the 'touch points' of the process (in this case, a difficult moment of truth when a patient comes to realise that he can't just go back to feeding his birds and putting his life at serious risk), and, together with input from the advisory group, enabled an interviewer's guide for patients (the next stage) to be compiled, and piloted and pre-tested with the patient members of the advisory group. In terms of the 'co' part of co-design it should therefore be noted that patients and staff not only participated in the later design of services (the intervention) but also in designing and evaluating the research methodology and approach for the project itself.

This period of observation of staff–patient–carer interactions was followed by wide-ranging and fairly unstructured interviews with a sample of the H & N staff, sometimes one-to-one, sometimes in pairs. We confidentially explored their perceptions of the service they were giving, and asked them what they thought the major touch points or critical moments were for patients and users in shaping their experience of the service. After the interviews and observation were completed and the issues shared initially with the clinical director of the service a feedback session for staff was organised (*see* Box B).

Box B: Description of the staff feedback event

We prepared a 25-page thematic analysis of the H & N service based on (a) our tape-recorded interviews with 12 staff members, and (b) our observations of the multi-disciplinary team meetings and fortnightly outpatient clinics.

The analysis first explored the wider organisational, management, and clinical challenges which the head and neck service was facing and the types of issues these raised (for example: issues that had arisen related to roles and structures, resources and systems, information and communications, and the culture of the clinic). We represented this latter issue in terms of the need for a shift as shown in Table B1.

Table B1 Shifting the culture 'from . . . to . . .'.

From . . .	To . . .
Strong H & N teamwork and co-operation	Whole micro-system integration (including patients)
Maintenance	Development
Short-term staff perspective	Longer-term improvement
Coping	Problem-solving and innovation
Fatalism	Empowerment and control
Doing/pragmatism	Learning/reflection/mindfulness

The analysis went on to briefly comment on the prevailing drivers for change that were likely to lend support to efforts to improve the patient and staff experience (for example, an external peer review of the H & N service was planned for later in the year and this would cover patient involvement within its remit). However, the bulk of the analysis was an examination – using direct quotations and fieldnotes – of the focal areas that the staff (and we, through our observations) had identified for improving the service and patient experience. Fourteen focal areas were described including, for example, the organisation of the multidisciplinary team meeting, patient experience of arriving and entering the outpatients clinic, how staff shared a diagnosis and provided information about the condition to patients, the insertion of the PEG feeding tube, managing the symbolic aspects of the illness and treatment, and various aspects of non-clinical services.

We fed this thematic analysis back to the clinical director of the head and neck service individually prior to sharing it with the wider staff group. The clinical director's response was:

> I mean there are no great surprises there. It [the clinic] is organised chaos fairly often and I think it's basically just grown without being re-organised and probably without a reassessment of 'can we actually deal with this number of patients in this amount of space and time?'. There are some constraints that we can't do anything about, like the size of the clinic, but there are some constraints that we can do things about, but need to sit back and look at them and in a sense re-organise. So, what we need to do is to do something about the things that we can do something about . . . We're looking for a group thing so we need to see what's wrong. We need to see what's right as well so we can build on it, but we need to be sensitive about the way we feed back and it's probably best coming from me.

A feedback session for all of the staff was then organised. The feedback was led by the clinical director himself using a set of PowerPoint slides summarising the key points in the analysis. The objectives of the session were to:

(a) feed back and validate the findings relating to staff experiences
(b) correct or add in anything that may have been missed out
(c) agree a two-column agenda of items: the first column consisting of issues they wished to carry forward to work on jointly with the other half of the co-design group (i.e. the patients), and the second of issues they preferred to work on separately (for example, the multi-disciplinary team (MDT) meeting), and
(d) gather suggestions about the design of co-design event with patients.

Following a lively group discussion of the focal areas from the thematic analysis, individual staff voted for what they perceived to be the most important issues. At the end of the staff feedback session six priorities were identified. These clustered around (in descending order of priority):

1   the post-surgical ward (with specific mention of how best to provide care for a wide casemix of patients, staff skills and training, and the 'mirror moment')
2   'knowing who is in each room' (in the outpatient clinic)
3   psychological care and depression
4   signposting
5   PEG policy
6   the waiting room (in the outpatient clinic).

Patients and carers

Observation and staff interviews were followed by interviews with 12 patient volunteers which took place either in their homes or the hospital, the choice of venue being theirs (on this occasion numbers were fairly evenly split). In this case all the interviews were filmed and tape-recorded with the patients' formal consent. Patients and carer interviewees, who were identified and recruited either directly by clinic staff or via a general poster displayed in the waiting room of the clinic, were sent a letter (signed by the researchers and local leaders of the hospital) explaining the purpose of the project. These letters were followed by face-to-face briefings and the signing of the required ethical protocols before the commencement of the interview. The letter also outlined the main headings of the ground to be covered so as to help the patients and carers begin the process of recalling and reflecting upon their experiences in advance of the interview. The interview guide (see Appendix 1) retained the rough chronology of events, allowing the interview to follow the course of a narrative or story: 'So, let's begin at the beginning' . . . 'What happened next?' . . . 'Can you remember how that felt at that point?' . . . 'If you went through that again what would make it easier/better for you?', so that it was the patient taking the researcher through every stage of his or her journey, as naturalistically as possible, and with minimal intervention from the interviewers. Although the interviewer may use the different stages of the journey as the organiser for the interview or conversation, the whole point of this process is that the teller is able to tell it exactly as he or she wants, at times freely jumping over and missing out large tracts of the journey, and at other times zooming in and concentrating on, what for others, might appear to be small details (which clearly are not).

Thus, patients and carers were more like teachers or guides than interviewees (*see* the earlier discussion in Chapters 4 and 8 of the role reversal that needs to occur in this kind of process). Predictably, they would sometimes completely pass over parts of their journey which we and staff had expected to be important, and at other times focus on things which to us seemed almost minor or trivial but which clearly had major symbolic significance for them. The stories, which in this case were by their choosing, always told by a duo of patient and carer (usually partner – cancer is very much a shared journey), concluded with a series of questions around particular themes and issues such as information, and level of involvement in choice of treatment, which are known to be important issues.[5] In many ways, the research method underpinning the initial stages of the EBD process was therefore no different from the host of narrative and storytelling methods currently deployed in healthcare and other organisational settings and described in earlier chapters.[6–8] The one significant difference from, say, the Discovery Interview was that the interview 'spine' for the stories and possible key themes and issues were initially identified and developed jointly by patients and staff as part of our commitment to co-design, so that everyone had full opportunity to comment on its form, language and content before going 'live'. Patients particularly were invaluable in pointing out errors, omissions or insensitivities in the line of questioning.

The material from the interviews, in this case in the form of a typed transcript and DVD, was shared with the participants to check they felt that it truly represented their experiences, and to stimulate any further reflections (which it invariably did). Seven patients took up our offer of using disposable cameras; particularly helpful were those that provided insight into the lives of the patients outside hospital (for example, the patients' role in maintaining and cleaning their neck valves). Two members of staff also took photographs of their daily work activities and routine.

After completing the 12 interviews, and analysing the transcripts and editing the films, a feedback event just for the patients and their partners/carers was organised. For the benefit of readers who would like to know more about the patient feedback event we describe it in detail in Box C.

Box C: Description of the patient feedback event

The patient feedback event was attended by seven patients and five carers, and held over the course of one day at a hotel conference centre. The designer on the project's core team had prepared clipboards with various materials and exercises for the day (for example, a 'review' sheet for the film of the patients' interviews and a grid of patient emotions identified from the patient interview transcripts – *see* Figures C1 and C2).

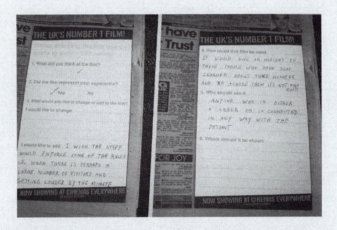

Figure C1 Film 'reviews'.

Emotional map

Anxiety	Fear	Happiness	Gloom	Despaired
Happy	Optimism	Shame	Out of control	Hope
Excitement Detachment	Envy Anger	Enthusiastic Confusion	Weepy Sick	No confidence Insecure
Apprehensive	Sadness	Exposes	Embarrassment	Hurried
Resentment	Pride	Powerless	Depressed	Unattached
Morbid	Guilt	Vulnerable	Fatalism	Shock
Hopeful	Numb	Powerless	Tearful	Self-loathing
Alone	In a pickle	Anxious	Lost	Annoyed

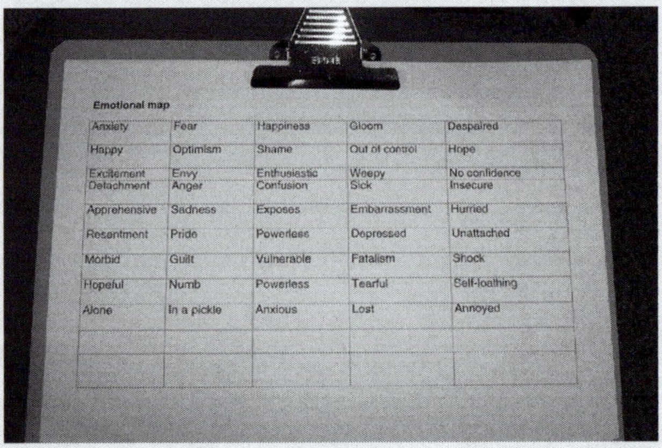

Figure C2 Patient emotions.

Before the patients and carers arrived we wrote the key stages of the patient journey (for example, diagnosis, surgery and discharge) along the top of a long sheet of brown paper hung on the wall. To this, we then added all the various touch points identified from the interviews (for example, waking up in ITU and radiotherapy planning). The day was facilitated jointly by the designer and service improvement practitioner from the core team.

We began the morning with a short 'icebreaker' and then invited one of the patients who was serving on the advisory group to say a few words about the aims and objectives of the day and his own role on the project. The film-maker on the core team then introduced the 35-minute film he had compiled from the patient interviews and other filming activities. The film was divided into seven chronological segments (for example, a montage of clips showing patients talking about when they noticed something was first wrong; a montage of clips showing patients talking about waking up in the intensive care unit (ICU)/high dependency unit (HDU) and the aftermath of surgery, etc.). The film was introduced in terms of showing 'your stories so far' and we acknowledged that there would be lots of important material from the interviews that had been edited out in the interests of time. The film was also intended to give the patients present an idea of how their individual experiences compared to other people's.

After the film was shown the facilitators explained that we wanted to use the film at the co-design event itself (i.e. to share the film with staff) and that we wanted the patients views on the film being used for this purpose. One patient commented that he found the film:

> *frightening . . . I want to move on now. If you want to frighten anyone then show them that [the film] . . . it's a good training aid but I wouldn't want to show it to someone who had just found she had cancer . . . It's an X-rated film. I wouldn't want to show it to my kids.*

We also asked the patients whether the film had the right things in it. Were there any other aspects of their experience they wanted to add in? Comments included:

> *[Patient A] thought a clip should be added about the lack of privacy on the post-surgical ward; he had been 'horrified to hear another patient being told he had terminal cancer on the ward'. [Patient A] also highlighted the importance of patient dignity on the ward and that there was a need for a day room. At one point he and his wife had wanted to play Scrabble and could only find a small room – more like a cupboard – so they settled down in there!*
>
> *[Patient B] thought there should be something on the film about the spiritual needs of patients: 'this should be brought out'.*
>
> *[Patient C] said he 'had been upset by visitors bringing their kids in with them . . . must be very disturbing for little children to have to see patients like us . . . I couldn't hide anywhere'. [Patient A] and his wife said that on this issue 'our 14-year-old son had to watch patients having their throats sucked out . . . it's more embarrassing, distressing for patients knowing that children are watching them'.*

> *[Patient B] also added that 'my biggest concern was MRSA [methicillin-resistant Staphylococcus aureus] and visitors not washing their hands, using toilets they shouldn't use . . . we've all got open wounds . . . need a bit of health and safety on that ward'.*

We then summed up before lunch by asking how we could bring all these important issues to life so that we can make changes. We asked the patients and carers, 'Do you have any other ideas about how you might like to share your stories with the staff other than through the film? What questions do you want to ask staff at the co-design event? How do you want to ask them?' Comments included:

> *[Patient B] said, 'I was glad to see the film because I was a bit frightened about how I sounded . . . it gave me a lot of confidence; I wasn't too bad. Did I really say that?!' Regarding the value of the interviews, [Patient B's carer] commented 'how helpful it is to be able to say so much, to have a captive audience with only a few prompts . . . for some individuals very therapeutic'. [Patient B] agreed: 'helpful in getting a sense of perspective . . . helps to get on with things'. [Patient A] said of the film that 'it can be seen and heard and doesn't lie . . . it can't be distorted. It wasn't embarrassing to do it; I just don't like watching myself . . . if it helps just one person to ease any fears . . .'. [Patient A's wife] commented that 'it was nice not to be sitting [when being interviewed] without a consultant or nurse again; it's about you, you're in control'. [Patient B's carer] added that 'this environment [in a hotel conference centre], not in the hospital environment . . . we're in control. Us being here and not there [in the hospital] is so important . . . all equal and individual . . . on a level playing field . . . all out of uniform'.*

After lunch the facilitators explained the key stages of the patient journey and the 'touch points' we had identified from the interviews and how we had sought to represent these (*see* Figure C3). The facilitators asked the patients to take five minutes and to move the touch points up and down a simple 'high'/'low' scale on the wall, identifying which touch points had been the best part (highlights) of their experiences and then the worst (lowlights). The facilitator noted that the patients might disagree among themselves about where to place each of the touch points (as their experiences of the same touch point may have been different) and that they could also add new ones to the map too if they wanted to. The result was an emotional rollercoaster revealing the highs and lows of their journeys, the emotional highs being recorded on post-its and posted above each touch point on the chart, and the lows posted below (*see* Figure C3). One patient laid one of her 'lows' on the floor – *see* towards the right of centre of Figure C3 – to show just how low she had felt at one particular point in time!

Having completed this exercise, the facilitator then asked the patients to take another five minutes to add to each touch point the emotions that they had felt at the time. (The emotions were derived from the interviews and were printed out on a grid – *see* Figure C2.) Again, the patients could add in additional emotions if they so wanted. So, for example (*see* Figure C4),

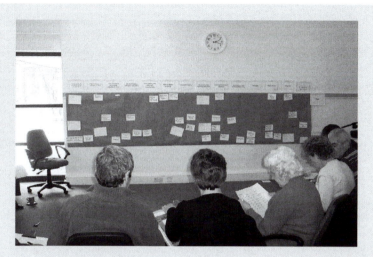

Figure C3   'Highs' and 'lows'.

at the first meeting with their consultant, patients chose to describe their emotions as 'numb', 'vulnerable', 'apprehensive' and 'powerless', and one patient added a new emotion expressing it in terms of 'I didn't know how to react to him or what to say' (far right of Figure C4).

The service improvement practitioner then gave a brief response to the completed experience map. It was a 'real rollercoaster' with some very positive touch points which we didn't want to design out of the service but rather affirm and explore why they were positive. The facilitator highlighted the issue of pain control which some of the patients had rated as a high point and others as a low point. Why were these different experiences?

> *[Patient A] had highlighted pain control as a positive: 'I had the choice . . . unless you talk to them they just assume you want morphine. I asked them questions and they said "it's your choice". And that was good . . . to be honest anytime you are in hospital and they give you a choice then that's a good point.' Other patients said that they had needed more information regarding pain control and to have been better informed. Others said that coming off pain control had been a problem, 'cold turkey . . . they overestimated our intelligence . . . nobody advised us.'*

The designer then explained the co-design approach (via a set of PowerPoint slides explaining the notions of 'co-design', 'touch points' and 'storytelling', and illustrating some of the tools for engagement we had used and were planning to use at the joint event). The group then broke out into small groups to discuss (as brief on slide): 'Which particular touch points we would like to discuss with staff at the co-design event, why we think each should be improved and our ideal solution (i.e. what should it be like, how can we reach this solution and who needs to be involved?).' The patients then broke into small groups and worked for 50 minutes on the sheets that the designer had prepared, producing their priorities for the forthcoming dialogue.

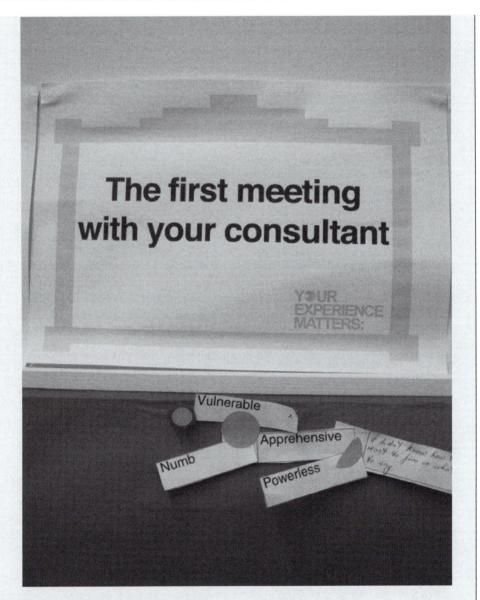

Figure C4 Emotional touch points.

Everyone then came back together for the final 45 minutes of the day to identify the six touch points that were felt to be the most important to address at the co-design event. After discussion led by the facilitators, and cross-referencing to (a) the results of the group work (on the completed worksheets) and (b) the experience map, six priorities were agreed:

1 post-surgical ward (with specific mention of staff training; privacy and dignity; spiritual needs)
2 'waiting for results'

3   information (about (a) condition; (b) hospital environment; (c) pain control)
4   radiotherapy unit (especially radiotherapy planning and the 'mask')
5   PEG
6   the outpatients clinic.

At the end of the day the patients were asked to spend a few moments reflecting on the day using 'Goodbye Sheets' the designer had prepared, and they were also offered some disposable camera packs to take away to capture anything else they felt reflected their experiences to date.

Co-design group meeting

This meeting represented the first coming together of staff and patients face-to-face to share their experiences of giving and receiving the service, using film and exercises to identify, agree and define key touch points where improvements might be made or the service strengthened. Box D details the format and content of the co-design day.

Box D: Description of the co-design group meeting

The co-design event was also held in a hotel conference room. Patients (and carers) and staff (surgeons, nurses, therapists, etc.) were invited to interview and introduce each other in pairs around the room. The sponsor of the project explained that the National Institute for Innovation and Improvement exists to find new ways to make the NHS a better place for patients. The Institute does this by testing new approaches in pilots that might then apply to the whole NHS; the EBD work with the head and neck service was one such pilot. She explained that no-one in the world is working in quite this way and, although this is just a test so far, everyone has been very positive about it. The information that has already come out is incredibly important in terms of developing a much better service: 'You are therefore pioneers of what we hope to see across the NHS.'

We then explained the EBD process we were piloting in more detail (using Figure 9.1 on page 120), detailing how the core group 'runs the work', and the advisory group is there to advise and steer but also to 'check us and makes sure we don't go off on some lunatic tangent, and advise us on leaflets and publications so they hit the spot'. We emphasised how the figure shows that both staff and patients are equally important; co-design is about bringing our learning and experience together, and asking 'what does all that mean', and 'what can we do to make the experience of the service better for both patients and staff?'. The aim of this co-design event was to form teams ('individual co-design groups') of patients and staff to help make changes and improvements to specific aspects of those experiences. We would then all come back together again in six months time to ask: have we made the changes? Have we improved the service? EBD was not just about talking but actually doing something.

One of the patient representatives on the advisory group then introduced the 35-minute patient film, saying that:

> *initially I was very apprehensive about the film but this and the interview transcript have turned out to be a double benefit. The transcript gave cause for further reflection on my experience but it was also a very therapeutic process. The film even more so, given that you are speaking to an emotionless camera.*

We asked patients and staff, as they watched the film, to think about the positive touch points but also the 'touch points that needed improving; to think of a particular area where you would be keen to start some work on'.

We then showed some photographs of the patient feedback day and briefed the staff on the issues and touch points that the patients had prioritised. The H & N clinical nurse specialist then provided a similar summary and update from the staff feedback day for the benefit of the patients. Following these updates we moved to some group work that aimed to put the staff and patient priorities together in a mind map of what we would like to work on from all the touch points that had been identified.

Individual co-design groups were formed around constellations of touch points (for example, there was a post-surgical ward group, a psychological support group, an outpatients clinic group). Patients and staff were able to put their name by any touch point they wanted to work on in the co-design process (*see* Figure D1).

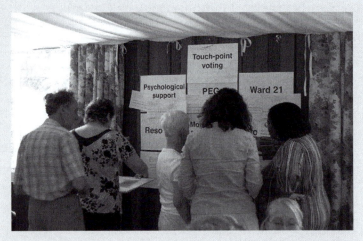

Figure D1   Agreeing priorities for improvement at the co-design meeting.

The groups then did some initial work on deriving some design principles around the touch points they had chosen to work on. We used a simple A4 sheet to ask the groups to think about how to improve patient and staff experiences using the formula: 'If you want to achieve Y in situation S, something like X might help' (*see* Chapter 7). As a result of the co-design day, six co-design groups were formed:

1   the post-surgical ward
2   psychological support

3   the radiotherapy unit
4   PEG
5   the outpatients clinic
6   carer support.

Details of the composition and ongoing work of the groups were posted on the project website which also allowed patients and staff to record their views of the process, details of upcoming meetings and updates of completed actions. We include a small selection of these postings below to illustrate how much energy and interest was generated by this first co-design day:

> *Hi everyone*
>
> *Wasn't it a pleasant and fruitful afternoon we had on 12 May? Thank you to all patients and carers for sharing your experience and identifying areas on which we can work together for the benefit of other patients. One particular issue that kept being raised was the importance of having accurate information regarding the planning of radiotherapy before getting to [hospital x]. We have already taken steps to address this – [the clinical nurse specialist] will ensure that all patients for radiotherapy will have written and verbal information on what to expect at their first planning appointment. We have 'helpful hints' leaflets at [hospital x] describing the making of the mask and the planning . . . We are also discussing the making of a video about radiotherapy planning . . . I will keep you informed as we progress.*
>
> *Good morning everyone*
> *We would like to thank everybody who came to the first meeting last Thursday and for sharing their or their family members' experience of PEG tube. We had a good meeting which started with the sharing of everyone's thoughts about PEG which had been set as homework! We asked: how they would describe their PEG . . . It was a good experience when . . . How would you rate your experience with PEG . . . scale running from Good to Bad . . . My experience was affected by . . . The story I tell about the PEG . . . and the word or emotion which best describes my PEG experience. Here are a few samples of comments made:*
>
>> *'I would describe my PEG as part of the care and concern by all the staff at the L & D hospital shown to me both pre-op and after my operation right to the day that it was removed . . .'*
>>
>> *'It was a good experience when I could rely on and have peace of mind in getting sustenance immediately following my operation and in the later stages of radiotherapy. At both times oral intake would have been near impossible . . .'*
>>
>> *The story that I tell about my PEG is . . . 'It was vital for my health but restricts your movements for long periods of the day; treatment and advice by hospital staff has been very good.'*
>>
>> *It was a good experience when . . . 'it wasn't a good experience at all . . .'*
>>
>> *The story I tell about PEG is . . . 'not to tuck the tube end in your knickers'. (Guess who!)*

The story I tell about PEG is . . . 'once or twice we forgot to close the clamp before flushing and connecting the food pipe and had the contents of my stomach everywhere!'

We discussed the whole journey before and after PEG insertion and continued feeding during treatments and rated specific touch points to identify positive or not so positive stages which affected each individual.

The areas which are not so positive are to be discussed at the next meeting to identify action to be taken if changes are feasible. Some changes to the services have already taken place regarding patient information about tube removal (sedation vs local anaesthetic spray).

Other areas for discussion at a further meeting includes: ward stay, choice in PEG dates, knowledge of staff, pain management, discharge, and drugs to take home.

We will be in touch soon with another date for another meeting. We would love to see you all again.

Just to let you all know a little about progress on [head and neck ward]. The admissions room can now be used in the evenings as a quieter place for patients and family to sit. The ward environment has been looked at and many posters taken down to increase the light into the bays. More work is planned to improve work areas by reducing clutter and to make sure items are stored closest to where they are needed.

The staff have tried a quiet time after lunch once or twice. Some patients welcomed this but one bay of ladies did not want to do this at all. Some of the ward staff have not yet had the chance to listen to the accounts of patients' experiences and so we have arranged for them to be able to do this next week. The ward staff have also started to look at various ways of bringing all ENT (ear, nose and throat, and head and neck) patients to ward 21.

A small group of staff and patients are devising a way of guiding the care needed on a day-to-day basis and reviewing the skills required to care for patients who have particular surgery, e.g. laryngectomy.

An action plan including the above has been devised and individual staff are signed up to their part of the plan. We have one or two 'patient' volunteers willing to be part of judging how well the work progresses by visiting in a few weeks. We would welcome other volunteers who would like to do this.

Hi all,

[x] and I thoroughly enjoyed the day on the 12th. We feel that it was really worthwhile. The following day I visited a new laryngectomy patient in hospital. He had undergone surgery the previous Monday and I had met him prior to surgery. He was in really good spirits and I am confident that he will be a willing 'recruit' on my 'crusade'. I told him that I would require his help when is a bit fitter and I think that he will be pleased to help.

In reply to [y's] comment re meeting up to discuss the PEG, I will be happy to join this discussion; I feel that I have something to offer to this aspect. I will try to be available whenever a date is decided on.

A few things have come to mind that we could be proactive in:

1 *Gaining knowledge and expertise of the benefits that might be available to laryngectomy patients and cares, such as Disability Living Allowance, Attendance Allowance, disabled parking badges, etc. This is something that we could perhaps consult the Macmillan service about. I know that the National Association of Laryngectomy Clubs has done some work in this area and could also be consulted.*

2 *Some time ago I read an article about an initiative in Belfast that involved training 'hospital visitors'. This was aimed at those offering support to people awaiting surgery and immediately after surgery. I think that there would be some merit in exploring this to try and establish if something along the same lines could be undertaken by the [hospital]. It need not be restricted to laryngectomy as the same principles would apply to a broad range of patients.*

I think that if the above mentioned subjects were to be undertaken new initiatives would spring from them. It could also be helpful if an experienced 'patient' were available to visit new patients at home to offer guidance with things such as the use of the feeding pump, for those new to the idea of a PEG. This sort of support could be, I think, offered once a rapport had developed between the new and the experienced patient.

That's all for now. I will continue to post, as new ideas will come to me as I continue along the road.

Best regards to you all.

Following this initial meeting of the co-design group, further 'individual co-design groups' (or 'touch-point groups') were established to deal with particular clusters of touch points around different parts of the service (for example, as happened in the case study, around the outpatients clinic, post-surgical ward, etc.) or types of issue (psychological support, carers, etc.). The advantages of this are that experiences can be delved into more deeply, and the net of participation extended to a wider group of people. During this implementation phase, members of the core group continued to draw on the data collected and worked with front-line staff and service users to implement a 'design' approach to each planned service improvement. Throughout, the focus remained on (a) using ethnographic storytelling, (b) experience- (user-) based mapping, (c) critical 'touch points', and (d) building a model of design rather than an abstract system of care. A user-friendly EBD website was also set up following the first co-design event to enable further exchanges of information and experiences between participants, providing both continuity of process and a means for sub-groups to keep in touch with and learn from each other, and the integrity of the 'whole' patient journey/experience preserved (see Box D). Later the individual co-design groups come together again (and this process can continue as long as necessary) to review and evaluate the improvements, and to celebrate their successes.

The identified priorities

Table 9.1 shows how the priorities identified separately by (a) staff and (b) patients were then finalised at (c) the co-design group.

As Table 9.1 illustrates, six separate individual co-design groups were formed following the initial co-design group meeting. Three of these groups (the post-surgical ward, PEG and the outpatient clinic) were entirely consistent with the priorities identified by both the staff and patients. The detailed action plans formulated by these three groups were also broadly consistent with the touch points identified from the original staff and patient interviews and subsequent co-design group discussions. Of the remaining three groups (psychological support, radiotherapy unit, and carer support), each emerged from the EBD process in differing ways. The 'psychological support' group formed around a combination of (a) what staff saw as a need for more extensive psychological support for patients with depression, and (b) many of the information touch points identified by patients. Interestingly, the use of the term 'psychological support' for this team was coined by patients not staff. The emphasis on the radiotherapy unit came very much from patients (as staff from the unit were only marginally involved in the EBD process which had taken as its primary focus the outpatient clinic at the hospital), and its emergence as a significant touch point raises an important question regarding the boundaries that are put around an EBD process. The final group – carer support – was not explicitly identified by the staff or patient fieldwork but rather emerged from discussions at the co-design event itself.

Regarding those priorities identified either by staff or patients that appear not to have been picked up at the co-design meeting, the touch points around the patient priority of 'waiting for results' is now part of the ongoing work of the

Table 9.1 Comparison of staff, patient and co-design group priorities.

Staff event (ranked in descending order)	Patient event (not ranked)	Project teams formed after co-design event
Post-surgical ward (casemix, staff skills, 'mirror moment')	Post-surgical ward (staff training; privacy and dignity; spiritual needs)	Post-surgical ward
–	'Waiting for results'	–
'Knowing who is in each room' (in clinic)	–	–
Psychological care and depression	Information (about (a) condition; (b) hospital environment; (c) pain control)	Psychological support
–	Radiotherapy unit (especially radiotherapy planning and the 'mask')	Radiotherapy unit
Signposting	–	–
PEG policy	PEG	PEG
Waiting room (clinic)	Outpatients clinic	Outpatients clinic
–	–	Carer support

'psychological support' group; the staff priority of 'knowing who is in each room' (in clinic) has been picked up by the outpatient clinic group; and the staff priority of 'signposting' is being dealt with as part of a wider hospital initiative. Therefore, as far as we are aware, nothing has been left out or forgotten.

At the time of writing the EBD process is still ongoing and work is underway to improve 43 specific 'experiences' across the groups. A further co-design event took place between staff and patients some five months after the initial co-design meeting in order to review and evaluate what had been achieved (*see* Chapter 10).

Touch points

The aim of the patient and staff interviews and observational work, both singly and in combination, was to help patients, carers and staff to identify and then jointly explore the many and various 'touch points' on their care or treatment journey, obviously with a view to designing better experiences around these. On the following pages we discuss the concept of touch points in a little more depth and illustrate their value in an EBD process by using examples that arose in the case study.

Touch points, which we have already mentioned briefly, represent the key moments or events that stand out for those involved as crucial to their experience of receiving or delivering the service. As described in Chapter 1, others prefer to use the term 'experience clues'.[9] Whichever term is used, these are the points of contact with the service that are the intensely 'personal' points on the journey, where one recalls being touched emotionally (feelings) or cognitively (deep and lasting memories) in some indelible kind of way. They are the points of emotional and cognitive connection, the 'big moments' – as an oncologist we interviewed called them – that patients and users will keep coming back to in the telling and retelling of their stories of care in the years following their treatment. Among the many articles that have been written about touch points (to the point that they have become something of a buzzword in today's design circles) Marty Gage and Preetham Kolari's seminal article 'Making emotional connections through participatory design' still offers one of the most accessible and practical introductions to the concept.[10]

This concept of identifying touch points is central to EBD. In the early days of the airlines they were referred to as the 'moments of truth', the crucial times when you call to make a reservation to take a flight or when you arrive at the check-in desk when your overall 'view' of the airline, good and bad, is formed,[11] whereas the less dramatic terms 'contact points' or 'critical points' are now the preferred choice of customer experience and customer management professionals.

Berry and colleagues[9] have also established a useful connection between touch points and 'experience' by referring to them as 'sub-experiences'. In the following they offer a definition of the term and an example:

> By 'sub-experience' we are referring to a specific experience that is part of the customer's overall experience with an organisation . . . The airline trip puts the traveller in at least three service 'factories': the departure airport, the airplane, and the arrival airport. Within each of these factories, the traveller experiences facilities, equipment, amenities, various service providers, and other customers. The airline trip involves a complex set of sub-experiences over a period of hours,

*with many opportunities for the traveller to be pleased, disappointed, or infu-
riated. In short, an airline trip involves a torrent of service experience clues –
clues that need to be managed.*

As we know, the 'health traveller' passes through service 'factories' (GP surgery, outpatients, inpatients, etc.) identical to those referred to here – usually
over a period of months rather than hours – encountering various kinds of sub-
experiences as they go, and just as the airline traveller's experience of the airline
is shaped and coloured by the accumulation of these sub-experiences, or even by
one or two that stand out above all (a rude staff member, a serious delay, wonderful cabin service), so too will the overall patient experience be shaped by their
sub-experiences in the GP's surgery, outpatient and inpatient factory.

There are few projects in healthcare that have used this touch-points approach
to service design but a recent exception, albeit covering only part of the journey,
was a pioneering and largely successful UK design industry–NHS demonstration
project, carried out in an Accident & Emergency (A&E) department and on-ward
in two hospitals. Staff and patient participants together with designers identified
six critical points relating to 'the most universal and emotion-laden moments in
the patients' experience', which on a wider scale the authors also claimed 'affect
large numbers of people and tend to colour their perception of the NHS generally'.[12] So, in the case of the A&E department, the 'arriving' critical point
included 'finding your way', 'the arrival area', 'security and privacy', and the
'registration' critical point included 'registering with dignity', 'feeling secure', and
'understanding the process.' On the basis of their detailed analysis and discussions, the design team was able to effect some impressive improvements that led
to physical changes in buildings, signage and spaces, including creation of a new
reception hub for patients, and other major changes.

Not to take away anything from the obvious success of this project, the only
questions one is left to ponder are whether perhaps too much emphasis was
placed on redesigning the physical environment and too little on the clinical
process and microsystem, and whether patients and carers were involved in the
team as fully-fledged co-designers or merely consulted by the professional
designers as the project unfolded. From an EBD designer's point of view, the
quality of the users' experience of a product or service is the sum of all their
interactions with that product or service, particularly those around the various
touch points (positive and negative) where the experience was at its 'hottest' or
most emotionally and cognitively intense. This does not mean that issues around
the physical environment were not raised by patients in the case study. For
example, one patient described how her bedside locker sometimes had a mind of
its own: 'none of the lockers had four castors that actually all rolled in the same
direction . . . you'd watch them rolling down the corridor!'

To retain balance in the argument, but always to be thinking of ways we might
improve the EBD process in future, we might suggest that if the A&E type case is
too focused upon the physical environment, 'touch points', as used in this case,
are too focused upon the psychological elements. Perhaps there is therefore
much to be gained by revisiting Hester's 'sacred places' methodology (*see* page
110), which undoubtedly shows a more even balance between the two.

The Joinedupdesignforhealth team[12] usefully describe the 'hot' experiences
referred to here as the 'chain' or 'necklace' of subjective experiences that make

up the patient and carer's journey, and that may be very different from the objective formal process map or clinical care pathway. Methods may vary but any touch-point analysis should always be striving to achieve what computer scientist David Gelertner, in his book *Mirror Worlds*,[13] called 'Topsight' – an informed vantage point that provides parallel insights into both the big picture (i.e. the necklace) and the way its component parts fit together to form the whole. We cannot stress how important it was that those involved were starting the design process from the same vantage point, and being on their guard from the very start against the danger of 'fragmenting experience'.

Returning to the case study, as Figures 9.2 and 9.3 make clear, it is a fairly straightforward task to reconcile the familiar objectively-based 'clinical process' map (Figure 9.2) found in the mainstream service redesign literature – and which to date has formed the basis of most healthcare service change/improvement interventions – with a subjectivity-based 'experiences map' based on touch points (the exemplar 'callouts' in Figure 9.3). Previously, we discussed how important it

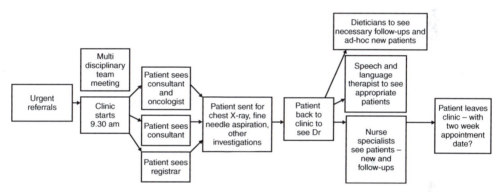

Figure 9.2 Traditional staff-led process map: head and neck outpatients clinic. *Source:* Head & Neck Combined Clinic, Process Map, 20 January 2003.

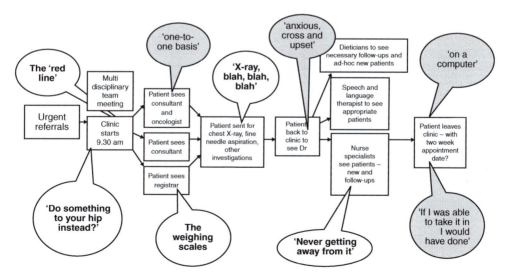

Figure 9.3 Patient experience map: head and neck outpatients clinic.

was to bring process redesign, governance and experience design together in one framework (Chapter 1), which we believe this graphic begins to help us to do. The traditional 'process map' in Figure 9.2 objectively charts, from left to right, the ideal steps in the first stage of the head and neck cancer patient's journey (namely their first attendance at an outpatient clinic), and is well suited to identifying problems and solutions, and finding ways of compressing or cutting out the cul-de-sacs and unnecessary steps on the journey. This is the familiar notion of process redesign which is especially well suited to dealing with the functionality and engineering aspects of the service (P and E).

In contrast, the staff, patient, and carers' stories as related in the interview conversations, supplemented by the observational data, revealed a dimension of care and treatment that is largely missing from the traditional process map; the third element in our overarching design model on page 5 (A). This missing dimension is the chain of experience or 'experience map' shown in Figure 9.3. Each of these 'callouts' represents an 'experience anecdote' that arose naturally in conversation, as patients and carers told their stories of receiving care and treatment. These came entirely from the tellers (emic, actor-centred as opposed to the etic, expert process maps – *see* earlier), and were neither anticipated nor predetermined in any way by the interviewer. Behind each 'callout' (and only a small number of those we were told are included in Figure 9.3) there was a story to tell – a story that would take in the whole range of emotions, good and bad, from wry humour, hope, optimism, security and relief to anger, fear, vulnerability, confusion and disbelief.

This subjective, actor-centred, existential focus is what differentiates experience mapping from more conventional process mapping, while recognising that good service design probably requires the synergies from using both. Others have also argued that care pathways and patient-centredness need not necessarily be dichotomous, even though they may often have been treated that way.[14]

What follows are four brief examples taken from the huge arsenal of patient and carers' touch-point stories that we gathered from interviews and direct observation of behaviour. Limitations of space prevent us from describing even the limited number of touch points shown in Figure 9.3 but the examples used (the white callouts in the figure) will hopefully serve to illustrate what a rich source of knowledge, guidance and insight these emotionally charged touch points can provide alongside the traditional 'process map' approach and within a broader design process.

'Do something to your hip instead?'

Our first anecdote begins with the all-too-common problem faced by patients of actually trying to find their way to the outpatient clinic; a task often hampered rather than helped by the signage in the hospital. In the case of the combined head and neck clinic that serves as the case study, patients were told to look for signs to 'ENT Children' and were then surprised – and a little unnerved – to find themselves sharing the clinic waiting area with orthopaedic outpatients:

> *For a start, it said something like, go along the corridor and what you had to look for then was ENT Children, and I thought, well, perhaps I'm reverting to childhood, but . . . so it was a little odd! Then it was extremely odd waiting in the clinic because there was also an orthopaedic clinic going on and later on,*

because that still happens, I did think to myself, 'I wonder what happens if you wander into the wrong clinic? Do they just do something to your hip instead?'

As we said earlier, there are funny stories, even in an H & N clinic!

The weighing scales

Before patients are taken through to the consultation rooms in the clinic they are asked to remove their shoes and to step on to a set of weighing scales. The scales are in a side corridor but in full view of everyone sitting in the clinic. One patient commented that:

> *I think that could be done in the consultant's room. It only takes seconds. I don't know why they have to weigh somebody before they go for their consultation . . . it only takes seconds, it would be in a much more private environment. Because you go in there in your ordinary clothes and you have to take your shoes off.*

We observed patients, either through age, frailty or obesity, who were unable to bend down to remove their shoes in full view of all the other patients sitting in the clinic. Just to add to their difficulties, 'there is nowhere to put your coat and shoes and things, and you're looking for somewhere to balance it all while you jump on'. The Medical Director's reaction to his patients' evident discomfort, and lack of privacy and dignity in this mundane setting, led him to say 'let's just move them [the weighing scales]'. This response illustrates how solutions to some of the issues identified in an EBD process can be implemented almost immediately; other touch points require longer-term solutions including, for example, the reallocation of resources or new staff roles. Given so many bad experiences around the weighing scales, it should also prompt those involved to query whether 'weigh patient' should even remain part of the traditional pathway, especially when patients were sometimes being weighed with jacket or shoes on and sometimes with them off, and told us that they were mostly monitoring their own weight at home anyway. One thing an experience focus can do is point out some of the 'mindlessness' around some of the routine activities embedded in a pathway

'X-ray, blah, blah, blah'

Once seen by a consultant in the clinic, patients would often be told that various further tests and investigations would need to be carried out. Some of these would be done on the same day but, in the case of the patient speaking below, the process by which and where the tests would be done was very unclear, hence contributing to another negative touch point and a bad set of experiences:

> *So I saw [the consultant surgeon] and he told me what he suspected and then he gave me a list of things I had to do that day. X-ray, blah, blah, blah. He asked me to wait outside and I would be called. I misunderstood what I had been told. I thought I had to go off and get the X-rays and the blood, so off we went looking for all these different departments and eventually we got everything done, you know the X-ray, the blood tests and a few other bits and bobs, and on the list was to go to Ward One. So eventually we went to Ward One and*

the nursing sister said what happened to you? We've being waiting an hour and a half for you. So I said no I've been getting all these tests done, and she said oh, you were supposed to come here first and then everything would have been done with the one stop shop, as it were. That had not been fully explained to me.

'Never getting away from it'

Our final example relates to the volume of letters and instructions sent or given out to patients by the various different departments involved with their treatment and care, and the number of occasions on which they were required to attend the hospital:

the frequency of the hospital visits, and I thought I would go mad because it seemed we were coming down here every day for one reason or another, very often at short notice. Sometimes twice a day, because we had to come down for my husband, and sometimes hospital appointments were altered at short notice. And you felt you were never getting away from it, because you would have come down here, there was a letter from them! . . . So I did feel at times I was going mad and I was out of control. I had to sort of stop and say, 'now calm down. They're pulling out all the stops. They're doing everything they can to help you.'

Of course, these stories and touch points continue beyond a patient's first attendance at the outpatient clinic and run for the whole of the care and treatment episode, often engendering stronger emotions than embarrassment or mild discomfort of the type caused by weighing scales. For instance, after surgery, patients would often have a short stay on the intensive care unit. There were touch points here, too, of course, and not just for patients – 'these machines were all making different noise, gurgling and bleeping and so on. My biggest concern [when I came round] was that I had a tube coming out of here and a bellow thing, with the noise it was making and I thought my lungs weren't operating, I was on some kind of life support system. That made me think things hadn't been quite as straightforward. That made we wonder. If you switch that off, will I be able to breathe?' – but also for carers visiting the unit:

But I have to say when I came into the intensive care unit I was very, very surprised. That was 1 March, it was cold and imagine coming in at 10 o'clock at night; it was fairly bleak. And they let me into the door and then into the visitor's room at the side and I'd got my big anorak thing on. And then they said 'we're just sorting him out, we'll call you in a few minutes'. And then they came and called me, no-one said, wash your hands, take your coat off, put a cloak on or anything. I did take my coat off as it happens . . . They didn't ask me to take off shoes, coat or anything. So I was amazed, absolutely amazed.

This latter quotation reinforces the importance of including carers in the EBD process and building the design around them as well as patients and staff.

Patients would then be moved to a ward, typically for a week or more. It became clear that this particular part of their experience typically contained several touch points which had a profound effect on their overall recollection of the interaction with the service. One of these was the patient's first experience of being 'high'!

> . . . and then suddenly the pain started to kick in. Wow! I'm allergic or I react to anything that's a codeine derivative, and I'd made this quite plain, but there wasn't anything else on offer to me at that time, other than paracetamol, headache pills! And I was eventually persuaded to have a minute dose of diamorphine. Wow! Never again! I hallucinated. My hand was a big octopus and I had to keep making sure they were on the bed. And I had this terrible moment of, like, nightmares and things, and I couldn't make anybody hear, because the locker was behind me and the bell was on it and this was in the early days when I was all trussed up with my drains. And there was no way, even if I'd been aware of it, I couldn't reach the bell. The night before I couldn't actually call loud enough, and even when a nurse was in the ward, my voice didn't seem loud enough to attract her, so I couldn't get any help, and then later on in the night, I got these chest pains and I could feel my chest getting tighter, and I eventually managed to attract some attention and she said, 'you should have rung the bell'. And I felt quite angry about it. And I was angry, too, because they said, 'the doctor's coming,' and no doctor came, and I said, 'please stay with me because I feel I'm going to die.' And I really did, because these chest pains were so bad and I was still hallucinating and I just wanted to know that I was still living and there was somebody with me. I think it was absolute terror.

And one further, probably quite familiar, example of a touch point on the ward:

> one morning, about five or six in the morning, I desperately needed to go to the toilet and I eventually got a nurse to come along and at this stage I was still wired up to machines and there were tubes coming out. And all I wanted was some means of getting to a little wheelchair or I could have pushed myself around on a frame, and I managed to communicate to this nurse that I needed to go to the toilet and she brought along a commode and just left me on this commode with no means of cleaning myself and I felt that was a very big shock to my dignity . . . She just walked away and left me and then I had to sit there for quite some time before anybody came along.

This experience of complete helplessness in the face of fear or loss of dignity is a good example of the kind of challenge a co-design group faces as it struggles to find ways of restoring control and peace of mind to the patient.

Finally, touch points would, of course, continue post-discharge as the following quotation from a patient story makes clear:

> I think your confidence takes a great knock. You don't know how people are going to react to . . . I mean, even now I wouldn't wander around the house uncovered in the neck because I think it might be upsetting for the others. I mean I'm okay with my wife, she's seen it from day one, but neither my sons nor daughters. I am aware of that and aware of their feelings. Same at work, if they had presentations then I'd volunteer to be the first one up to do the presentations, speak to large groups of people. I found that has changed, I don't put myself as forward as much because of my voice limitations and also because, as you know when you're doing a presentation it's very important to get the attention of your audience. Socially I find it quite difficult at times if I'm

in an atmosphere where there's lots of background noise and I can't make myself heard; I find that frustrating because I like to be heard. Little things. I can't whisper. Social niceties, if I'm on a train and I want to go to the toilet, I can't say 'excuse me sir'; I have to push people aside. I like to be courteous. Little things like that, the confidence is still a bit of a problem I must say.

Armed with both traditional process 'boxes' and experience 'callouts' (and the poignant, touching – often devastating – stories the latter contain), service designers, staff and patient, can begin to explore areas where improvements might be made, constantly switching between the objective (etic, outside in) and the subjective (emic, inside out) journey representations, and testing among other things whether a change to the first might help effect an improvement to the second, or whether a change to the second may require some kind of change to the first. In this regard, the stories contain all of the information designers are likely to require for the design process, and probably more besides. As the extracts show, they can refer to interactions with staff, the various steps in the journey, clinical procedures or the physical and cultural environment. With regard to the latter, for example, two patients mentioned the lack of attention paid to their spiritual needs, very reminiscent of one of Randolph Hester's 'sacred' places that had now become a 'sacked' place but which with a little imagination could soon be returned to the sacred:

> *I think I would like to add that the chapel at Hospital X is very crowded and it's so sad because it is meant to be used by everybody and every religion, but because it's small and on a Sunday I suppose they do have a reasonable number of people wanting to use it, so it has rows of chairs and I used to go in there sometimes on my way in or out and often would see one of the receptionists from the clinic who is a Muslim with her prayer mat and she had to put it down in the aisle. And when we came in she was always conscious that maybe she was in the way. And it would be so easy to leave enough room for Muslims to be able to put their prayer mat somewhere appropriate and comfortable for them. And the other thing was that it was right opposite an office where people went in and out all the time and there was loud chat. You could close the door, of course, if you wanted to, but that's not very welcoming always for other people. And so . . . I never found where the chapel was in Hospital Y, and the one I found in Hospital X was somewhere like it wasn't cared for and it wasn't recognised that there are people who would very much value that facility, and it could have been just that little bit better with just a little bit more thought.*

Our earlier point about bringing physical and symbolic design together in a single integrated process is thus well made here.

Just as people can be oblivious to some of the big things, so too can small things (at least to the outsider) acquire a disproportionately greater significance in the totality of experience, referring to things that do not even show up on the 'ideal' process map (a symbol literally being a mundane event or object that acquires a positive, 'more than' quality) as in the following four examples which also illustrate how touch points can be about good experiences as well as bad:

> *Yes, that was a big moment. I think I was still in intensive care, I think it was the second day and [the speech therapist] had come along and introduced herself.*

She held my hand. That was a big moment. And it wasn't patronising; it was just a professional thing. My hand was lying over the side of the bed and she took my hand and that gave me a wonderful message. And she said something along the lines of 'I know you've got worries at the moment and it's quite natural to have those worries but we'll all be working together on this and you'll speak again', that sort of thing. 'We'll get you speaking again.'

Everybody supported me very well. I won't name the names, but there was the neck nurse and she was tremendous. There was the lady who looked after my PEG and she was wonderful. And eventually . . . one thing I haven't mentioned, of course, my valve and my speaking, and the young lady who you all know, she's done a tremendous job in getting me to speak. We ended up reading poetry together which I'd like to do, and I found that the best way of learning to speak was through poems, and she trained me . . .

an old lady [the elderly volunteer at the information centre] who looked after me was 78 but she was like a spring chicken . . . she treated me like her son with cups of tea and little cakes.

I just wanted to record how incredibly helpful the people were from the moment we went to [the clinic], and there wasn't anyone who wasn't positive. And the Max Fax part of the scene was absolutely . . . you know, it was so sharp and so good, and I could hardly believe it when [the consultant] said that he would ring me that night when the operation was over to tell me how it had gone. And it seems so unlikely when one hears so much about the National Health Service, that the consultant was going to do that. However, he did and recorded that it had been a technical success and furthermore gave advice, you know, said, 'don't come in tomorrow until late in the afternoon, ring the ITU first, they'll advise you as to when [your friend] will be conscious', so I followed the advice.

On the negative side, the wrong word or look, or an unfortunate interaction with a member of staff, can be decisive. Clearly, the following is another wonderful example of the positive side, where a simple word said at the right time can literally transform a patient's experience:

While I was in hospital, I thought the care that I received from the team was wonderful because it was very painful and I had my moments of misery, but I wasn't allowed to feel miserable. We don't have miseries here! I felt that all the time people were sort of stretching out like hands, saying, 'come on. You're doing well. You're getting there', and everyone was gunning for me with such kindness, right down to the most junior member of the team to the senior member of the team. And I can't speak too highly of the team. And [the surgeon's] parting words were, 'Alison, you came in as a friend needing treatment, not as a patient with an illness'. And I thought that summed up the man. And I will always remember that and how much time he gave me and all the questions that he was prepared to answer to make sure I was satisfied and my husband was satisfied.

All of these examples give strong reinforcement to the point made in the opening chapter of this book that, unlike performance (P) and engineering (E), it is the aesthetics of experience (A), and close attention to them, that really makes the difference between *meeting* users' expectations and *exceeding* them. We can now see that the explanation lies in the 'more than' quality that comes from a well-managed piece of symbolic activity – a smile, gesture of kindness or friendship, or loving word – against which physical or systems issues may pale into insignificance.

This also applies to language and script which often are more important to the experience than either physical environment or setting, and can form positive experiences as well as negative. To take an example highlighted in Figure 9.3: how does the surgeon actually tell the patient he or she has cancer? How does the surgeon address this crucial 'management of information' issue? The communication issues surrounding a diagnosis of cancer are a rich and well-documented field for study. For example, Thorne and colleagues[5] interviewed 200 cancer patients to explore the impact of numerical information within cancer care communications from the patient perspective. The authors illustrate how numerical information has considerable potency for shaping the cancer experience, particularly in relation to feelings of hope, as well as offering a perspective from which to interpret issues of compassion, caring and informed consent.

In the case study, the patients told us that the words that are used in this exchange – the 'breaking the bad news' moment or touch point – are far more important than where the news is relayed, or even what is communicated (echoing our earlier point that the issue is not communication but information management and 'symbolic management' through the most powerful symbol of all: words). As part of our early observational work, described earlier in this chapter, we sat in on over 50 patient–doctor consultations and scribbled down the words used by the doctors during this crucial touch point. The words included: 'blisters', 'lumps', 'ulcers', 'polyp', 'warty things', 'necrosis', 'lesions', 'naughty tumour', 'aggressive', 'progressing', 'carcinoma', 'precancerous change' and finally 'cancer' itself. This variation prompted us to consider what the choice of language implied for the patients' experience at this key moment. Did the language used in fact matter? And why was there such variation anyway? As the patients told us subsequently this choice of words as well as the pace at which information is disclosed and style of their delivery did matter a great deal (*see* example below).

Four touch point scenarios

Of course, in all of this the fact that it is co-design – that patients are there in person, sat down with staff and designers, relating and discussing their stories and how it 'feels' to be in them – is what gives the design process its power, poignancy and, above all, impact. This is where the EBD process differs from much of what currently happens in healthcare, where as we have already noted patient stories are recorded in a studio and posted on a website or even read out by a third party in the design process (as is often the case with Discovery Interviews, for example). In itself, this may be an effective way of sharing experiences and enabling others to benefit from them, but it is not co-design because there is no design process as such. There is no live exchange or interaction, no joint sense-making, no process of moving from talk to action. Including users' stories and experiences in the design process may be one thing, but having users there in person and directly involved in examining and offering interpretations of their own experiences within the design process itself is really quite another. It does not just stop here: further power and weight may be added to the co-design process when not only the narrative voice of the patient and user are heard, but juxtaposed with the voice from the 'other side' – that of the staff member. The result is two, often very different, cross-cutting 'takes' on the big moments which *demand* some kind of synthesis or resolution, and which provide the co-design process with its energy and forward momentum

The first of four scenarios which we found in our data was where both patient and staff member identify and corroborate a touch point where improvements to patient experience could and need to be made. As an illustration, consider one of the most critical touch points in the case of a cancer patient: the point we have already briefly referred to when they are told for the first time that they have cancer, a moment which – as James relates[15] – generates 'disbelief, fear, lies and chaos' on a deeply personal level. Our research with such patients leaves us in no doubt that the words and manner in which they are told becomes etched on the memory as deeply as a signature cut into the bark of a tree – and both 'sides' know that, as they also know that there is always scope for improvement here.

> **The patient**: *I was able to take it in. I think I went into automatic mode of, 'okay, yeah, right. So it's cancer, what do we do now? What happens tomorrow? What's going to happen next week? How do we cure this? Let's get on with it.' With hindsight, I look back, and think, the way it was done, not on a personal basis, it was quite a professional, business-like: we've got the results, it is bad news, I'm going to hand you over to Mr X [surgeon]; he'll talk you through it. But that's personalities, and I'd never criticise people for it. Everybody's got their own personality, and there's nothing malicious about it, he's just a professional guy, so he does it his way. Everybody does things their own way, but I would have done it differently.*

> **The oncologist**: *I think probably the first critical moment is breaking the bad news. I still think that we're not doing that as well as it could be done. I have really very big issues about that . . . I think patients need a lot more time when they're having treatment options discussed and they are pretty well supported through that bit of it but there are not enough clinical nurse specialists to be, you know, we might be breaking news to three or four patients at the same time and the clinical nurse specialist can only be in one room at any one time so we could organise the clinic better, I think, for patients . . . The diagnosis, the treatment options discussion, those are very defining moments so I think we could organise the clinic better so that we don't have three or four people being told bad news and having treatment options all discussed at the same time . . . I think we need to train everybody to break it a bit better. I don't think I am in any way perfect at doing it, I know I'm not very good at doing it, but at least I've had some training on how to do it.*

In this case, both patient and oncologist clearly agreed that this is one touch point that needs to be addressed in the department's experience design process, as is the second example when the patients first see themselves in the mirror post-surgery and assess the extent of their disfigurement (the so-called 'mirror moment'):

> *. . . I don't think I really saw myself. I don't know if there was a mirror at the wash basin the other side of the room, but I never went near there to begin*

with, because there wasn't enough room really. So I used to go to those wash rooms which children could see in, and they don't encourage you to linger. They're dark and I suppose I didn't really like them, and I'm not sure whether there was even a mirror there. When I saw a mirror, I just sort of looked very quickly and didn't bother.

Staff also drew attention to this as a critical, potentially traumatic, moment for cancer patients, confessing that while the formal practice required a member of staff to be present at this first viewing, this did not always happen, usually because of staff shortages and heavy workload. On some occasions, because of this, patients had been found collapsed on the floor, and in shock.

Equally of interest, however, are three other scenarios, namely:

- touch points identified by patients and carers which have never been seen as such by staff, and which therefore come as a complete surprise to them when revealed
- touch points identified by staff that turn out not to be touch points for patients at all, again often to the surprise of staff
- touch points that are visible to staff but not to patients.

One example of a touch point identified by patients that later came as a surprise to staff was their lack of preparation and understanding of what the term 'radiotherapy planning' might entail. Although one staff member said to us that 'I think going through the planning process is very difficult but we go to great lengths to explain what's involved', the patient perspective was very different:

And she told us about the process of radiotherapy and wrote down on a very useful leaflet that she gave me, six and a half weeks Monday/Friday radiotherapy, planning beforehand and that I would need what she called a shell and I would call the mask, and I think I probably had to wait about five weeks before the planning began, but what I didn't realise was that 'planning' is nothing to do with sitting around a table discussing this. It's being done to and that was only disconcerting, but it was probably one of the worst periods. So we went down to [the radiotherapy centre] for the first planning meeting and sat outside this room which had red lights flashing on and off. We waited about half an hour because there was somebody else in there, and I did wonder why there were red lights and I still thought I was actually going to be discussing something with someone. So when I was called in there was a nurse whom I didn't see immediately, a female nurse, but the person I saw, somebody called Adam . . . I'm sure he won't mind me mentioning his name, came and said 'hello' and his name was Adam and said, right, strip to the waist, and I was absolutely dumbfounded because I simply didn't expect that this was anything to do with an examination or whatever. And I can remember the nurse, when I was on the couch, trying to pass me some stiff paper to put over the top of me and, of course, it wouldn't stay on anyway and looking back it was probably quite amusing, but at the time it wasn't really. And I know that somebody else actually said something to Adam and he said, 'well, I'm so used to it' and of course he is, but we aren't.

A further example of what staff would view as an unexpected touch point was the PEG tube surgically inserted into the patient's stomach to allow liquid feeding, which, though a small minor procedure compared to the major surgery they have already had on their head or neck, is a major touch point for them, occurring just at a point when the patient thought they were out of the woods:

> *Now they can take this PEG out like yesterday, because I'm not happy using it. At worst it's been very, very painful, far worse than I'd experienced really up here when I thought about it, when I got used to the nought to ten scale, and at the best it's been painfully uncomfortable and remains so. And it's been in four or five weeks now, and I have the prospects of having it [unclear] and maybe hopefully not the end of April. And it's really been the worst bit of the whole lot.*
>
> *... it was like a whale caught on the end of a fishing line ... next to the [radiotherapy] mask that was the worst experience.*

An example of the third scenario – a touch point for staff that turns out not to be a touch point for patient – was widespread staff anticipation (as reported to us) that the cramped and crowded conditions of the fortnightly outpatient clinic, and the long waits therein, would be a major negative touch point for patients. The analogy we drew in our feedback to staff regarding the organisation of the clinic was with the Shibuya pedestrian crossing in Tokyo which is reportedly the world's busiest. Located in front of Shibuya Station the crossing uses a four-way stop to allow pedestrians to inundate the entire intersection; it involves massive volumes of people going in many different directions – but it does work; people cross safely and miraculously rarely collide. The staff view of the outpatient clinic, by contrast was: 'It's bloody chaos.' Staff were therefore most surprised to discover that, while being a source of irritation to patients, such issues were not a major touch point; indeed the patients told us that even though a new clinic would be nice, they did not believe it would dramatically alter their experience of the service (another warning of the dangers of doing physical design without experience design).

Finally, an example of a touch point visible to staff but not to patients would be the multidisciplinary team (MDT) meeting that preceded each fortnightly clinic (which we sat in on and observed on a number of occasions). Patients were mostly unaware that this meeting, which involved case discussion of treatment options for each of the new patients to be seen in the clinic later that morning, even took place; nonetheless it was still a key moment in terms of decision-making with regard to each patient's future management and care, and one that would shape the patient's experience for months to come.

Insights from touch-point analysis

For those involved, the rewards of a systematic and careful touch-point analysis such as the one outlined above are (we believe) process insights at two levels, each contributing to the dynamism of the change intervention itself in its own distinct way: first, insights about specific experiences that left an indelible memory or trace in the patient's heart or mind, positive or negative, these being the specific targets to which the EBD change process can be directed; and, second, insights about the whole experience of care, in its totality from beginning to end – the 'chain' of experience.

Regarding this latter point, in our work on EBD we have been struck by what is, or should be, an obvious fact, namely that individual members of staff only see a small part of the whole patient's care or treatment experience; the part with which they are directly involved. The dangers – and challenges – of this are that surgeons, for example, see the cancer patient for diagnosis and surgery, and then may 'lose' them for months while they undergo radiotherapy or chemotherapy treatment in a different part of the hospital or even at a different hospital. When they see that patient again, in experience as well as clinical terms, this is a very different patient from the one they saw some months earlier, and yet they may not fully appreciate or take this into account in the ensuing service they give. As a cancer oncologist put it to us:

> By the time I return them to our partner hospital, they are pretty much 75% over what's gone on here, so nobody there, none of the staff, sees how the patients are when they're at their lowest and at their most unwell here. Likewise, I don't see them on the ward usually, sometimes I see them on the ward if I'm seeing somebody else and I'll say hello to them, but I don't see them when they're in the midst of the surgical procedures and recovering from that so there's a huge experience that goes on here that really the other hospital are not that aware of. Patients are much better by the time they get back there.

Handovers, themselves the cause of a good deal of comment and criticism in healthcare, are therefore not just a 'systems' matter but also (and this is rarely brought out in the literature) a 'continuity of experience' matter, and to this extent they will only begin to be improved when staff are in a position of being able to appreciate the patient experience as a whole. In other words, and strange as it may seem, staff have to find a way not only of handing over information about the patient, but handing over their experience as well. 'Joined-up experiences' is an unfortunate cliché but this should not detract from the enormous difference this would make to the quality of patient care, and EBD would be the obvious choice of mechanism for accomplishing this.

Design principles

In Chapter 7 we discussed the notion of design principles. These principles are the imperatives and 'must do's distilled from experience and practice which enable one to say: 'If you want to achieve outcome Y (for example, improving the patient experience) in situation S (attending an outpatient clinic), something like X (preserving patient dignity by moving the weighing scales) might help' (Romme as cited by Plsek and colleagues[16]). Viewed as design principles rather than behavioural rules the emphasis moves from a mindset of control (which many rightly perceive in negative terms) to knowledge, positive learning and evidence about what has worked, and more importantly why and how it has worked in the way that it has.

The long list of touch points collated from our data provides a description of patient (and staff) experience, but it is still only a *description*. In order to improve services we then needed to move to *prescription*, and from diagnosis to action in order to find the practical 'must do's, the imperatives, that would improve the user's experience of the service. To this end the next stage of the EBD process (and part of the co-design meeting described earlier in this chapter – *see* Box D) was to move to discovering the design patterns or principles that, should they be implemented, would bring about such an outcome. The tool used by patient and staff in the co-design meeting is shown in Figure 9.4. The role of the design principle is to show the broad path that needs to be followed in order to translate a 'touch point' into an 'action point' and to convert the identified problem or opportunity into a solution.

Based on the case study, we have found that we can indeed extract design patterns – and equally important, anti-patterns (*see* Chapter 7) – from rich narrative, as we can also help patients and staff themselves to derive them from focused discussion around the touch points as part of the EBD process (usually following identification and agreement of the main touch points). Taking our earlier touch point of the patient feeling confused about what 'radiotherapy planning' entailed, we could frame our joint search for a design rule around this part of the patient journey in terms of 'If you want to improve the patient experience of receiving radiotherapy treatment (Y) in the regional cancer centre (S), something like X might help.' This is also where we need to be on guard against the anti-pattern. We might upon first examination of the touch point quoted earlier, for example, deduce that one design principle (or X) might be 'always ensure that the patient knows what is coming next'. However, when we showed the films of the patient interviews to all the patients as a group it was clear that this seemingly common-sense design principle might have a very negative effect on patient experience. After viewing the films for the first time one patient said that:

> I took it [my cancer] as a [horse race] . . . take it one jump at a time, coming up to the [next fence], up and over, little hurdles . . . I gathered strength after every hurdle to go to the next one . . . If I had known I had a 20 foot jump right at the end I would have laid down.

In other words, for him at least, telling him everything would have led him to give up at the first hurdle. Beyond the specific, immediate response of 'let's tell them everything' to the acknowledgement that patients do not always know or understand what is the next stage in their treatment, the actual 'meta' design rule turns out – from discussions with this group of patients at least (it may differ for other groups) – to 'never do anything that might take away from the resilience and motivation of the patient'.

The 'radiotherapy planning' touch point is a clear example of why patients and staff need to interact on an ongoing basis in order to challenge the 'common sense' and ensure that any 'obvious' solutions are in fact the right or best ones, and not seductive anti-patterns posing as wisdom or statements of the obvious. It also shows that one cannot run a complex process, like care, 'by design principle'. The two principles in this case of 'tell them everything' (based on the logic that we should never deceive patients or keep them in the dark about their own illness) and 'preserve maximum patient resilience' are tramlines, boundaries or polarities that need to be managed and within which subjective judgements and difficult decisions will always need to be made. However, as the field of building architecture reminds us, while buildings cannot be built

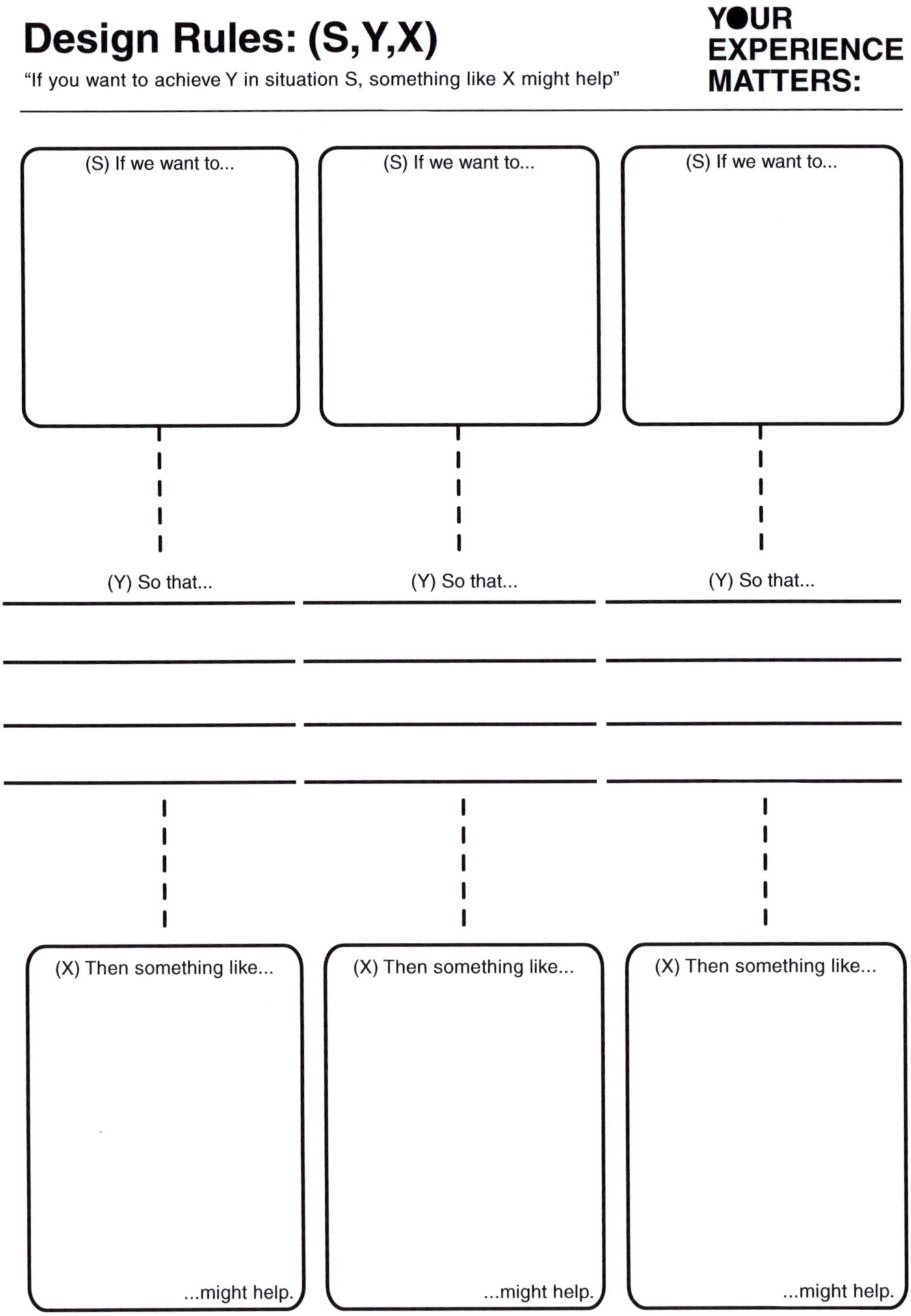

Design Rules: (S,Y,X)

"If you want to achieve Y in situation S, something like X might help"

Y●UR EXPERIENCE MATTERS:

(S) If we want to...

(S) If we want to...

(S) If we want to...

(Y) So that...

(Y) So that...

(Y) So that...

(X) Then something like...

(X) Then something like...

(X) Then something like...

...might help.

...might help.

...might help.

Figure 9.4   Deriving design principles.

solely by design principle, they will nevertheless fall down if the crucial design principles are not followed.

Taking stock

At the time of writing, one month after the second co-design event, staff and patients are continuing to meet and work together on the touch-point areas with the aim of improving a total of 43 jointly identified and agreed patient experiences. Many of the individual co-design groups have continued to 'recruit' new patients and carers, thereby broadening the experiences upon which the group can draw to identify and improve touch points. Members of the core team meet regularly with the chief executive of the hospital to (a) ensure that the ongoing work is integrated into the wider improvement efforts of the organisation, and (b) anchor the identified priorities into the performance management systems in the hospital.

As well as these specific pieces of activity, the improvement specialist from the hospital, who is a vital member of the project core team and the one closest to the day-to-day EBD process, views the 'general effects of the work' to date as being that:[17]

- The staff are less willing to wait for improvements (for example, in terms of patient information leaflets from the local cancer network) and more likely to want to fix it sooner themselves.
- There is greater confidence among staff working with patients in redesign activities.
- There is evidence of staff and patients increasingly looking outside their own service/locality for material from elsewhere to suit their purpose (for example, tracheotomy competency workbook and guidelines, patient instructions for crisis situations).
- Improvement has now spread to other areas (for example, to other parts of outpatients within the hospital).
- There is continued interest in and discussion about the work, even four months on (for example, the maxillo-facial consultants are requesting further opportunities to view the patient films and a discussion session about patient experiences, and the radiotherapy centre is very keen to use EBD as well).
- The ongoing process is becoming more self-managing in taking the improvement work forward.
- Staff are feeling that although they have tried unsuccessfully to improve some of these things before (for example, patient throughput in the clinic), this time they are actually managing to do so
- Patients are talking to each other in clinic about the work and making contact with each other and with staff by email and telephone, thereby generating a 'community' feel around the work.

Going beyond a straightforward description of the case study and the type of subjective assessment outlined above, the following chapter discusses various options for evaluating the impact of an EBD approach more formally, presents our own summative evaluation (using interviews with staff and patients), and also includes the reflections of our core team on how we might improve the approach next time.

References

1 Ussher J, Kirsten L, Butow P *et al.* What do cancer support groups provide which other supportive relationships do not? The experience of peer support groups for people with cancer. *Social Science and Medicine.* 2006; **62**(10): 2565–76.

2 Bate SP, Robert G. Towards more user-centric organisational development: lessons from a case study of experience-based design. *Journal of Applied Behavioral Science.* 2007; **43**(1): 41–66.

3 Erickson T, Smith DN, Kellog WA *et al.* Socially translucent systems: social proxies, persistent conversation, and the design of 'babble'. Proceedings of the SIGCHI Conference on Human Factors in Computing Systems; 1999 May; Pittsburgh, US. p. 72–9.

4 Bradner E, Kellogg WA, Erickson T. The adoption and use of 'babble': a field study of chat in the workplace. Proceedings of the European Conference on Computer-Supported Collaborative Work (ECSCW); 1999, September.

5 Thorne S, Hislop TG, Kuo M *et al.* Hope and probability: patient perspectives of the meaning of numerical information in cancer communication. *Qualitative Health Research.* 2006; **16**(3): 318–36.

6 Cortazzi M. Narrative analysis. In: Atkinson P, Coffey A, Delamont S *et al.*, editors. *Handbook of Ethnography.* London: Sage; 2001.

7 Bate SP. The role of stories and storytelling in organisational change efforts: the anthropology of an intervention in a UK hospital. *Intervention. Journal of Culture, Organisation and Management.* 2004; **1**(1): 27–42.

8 Greenhalgh T, Russell J, Swinglehurst D. Narrative methods in quality improvement research. *Qual Saf Health Care.* 2005; **14**: 443–9.

9 Berry LL, Wall EA, Carbone LP. Service clues and customer assessment of the service experience: lessons from marketing. *Academy of Management Perspectives.* 2006; **20**(2): 43–57.

10 Gage M, Kolari P. Making emotional connections through participatory design. *Boxes and Arrows.* 2000; 3 November. Also available on: www.boxesandarrows.com/view/making_emotional_connections_through_participatory_design (accessed 7 December 2006).

11 Carlzon J. *Moments of Truth. New Strategies for Today's Customer-Driven Economy.* New York: Harper & Row; 1987.

12 Joinedupdesignforhealth. *Critical Points. Improving Patient Experience of the NHS Through Design Interventions. Demonstration Project.* A report for the Sorrell Foundation in collaboration with Atelier Works, Fletcher Priest Architects, and Priestman Goode. London: Joinedupdesignforhealth; 2005.

13 Gelertner D. *Mirror Worlds: Or the Day Software Puts the Universe in a Shoebox: How It Will Happen and What It Will Mean.* New York: Oxford University Press; 1992.

14 Zuiderent T, Bal R, Berg M. *Patients and Their Problems: Dutch Alliances of Patient-Centred Care and Pathway Development.* Unpublished manuscript.

15 James N. Divisions of emotional labour: disclosure and cancer. In: Fineman S, editor. *Emotion in Organizations.* London; Sage, 1993.

16 Plsek P, Bibby J, Whitby E. Design rules grounded in the experience of managers: a system for organizational learning and pilot study of practical methods. *Journal of Applied Behavioral Science.* 2007; **43**(1): 153–70.

17 Hide E. *Progress Report: Experience-Based Co-Design of Head and Neck Cancer Services.* Internal project team report. 3 September 2006

Evaluating patient experience and experience-based design (and a brief word about patient satisfaction surveys . . .)

The overriding issue . . . is that although patients have been involved in one way or another with their own health, or the health of their friends, family or loved ones, their views and experiences may not have always been sought or indeed, their voices heard. With the many reforms that are coming on stream such as patient choice and practice based commissioning, it is essential that systems are put in place to ensure that views and preferences of patients and the public are listened to and incorporated into the planning, design and delivery of current and future services. (Department of Health)

Evaluating your EBD intervention

If you can't measure the impact you can't defend the value.

As the above quotation indicates, it is important to be able to evaluate the impact and success of your EBD intervention in some way (just like any other form of intervention) in order to decide whether it really was worth doing and worth repeating and spreading. This is particularly the case in a field like customer experience where organisational self-delusion, including healthcare, is an occupational hazard, and where staff – often egged on by glowing patient satisfaction surveys (*see* later) – are quite certain that they are already providing excellent service and an excellent experience for their customers, so why bother with EBD at all? In this regard a recent survey (cited by Allen and colleagues[1]) is salutary, revealing just how commonly companies misread their market. They surveyed 362 firms and found that 80% believed they delivered a 'superior experience' to their customers. But when they asked customers about their own perceptions, they found that they rated only 8% of companies as truly delivering a superior experience. Our only comment on this issue is that we should not assume self-deception on this scale to be the sole prerogative of the private sector!

In regard to evaluation, 'success' may be measured in terms of 'subjective' outcomes (for example, the way patients feel – our old friend A or aesthetics of experience), 'objective' outcomes (for example, reduced waiting times, fewer critical incidents, i.e. P performance and E safety and reliability), and in relation to any number of dimensions: personal, social, financial, environmental or ethical. Methods may also range from formal quantitative measurement to informal qualitative feedback. There is no single best way among these many alternatives that can be recommended, except to say that final choice of method needs to be guided by the three well-known precepts of evaluation:

- be able to answer what you think 'success' will look like and how you will know when you have got 'there'
- 'understand what matters, measure what matters, change what matters'; in other words, assess against what was considered important to achieve at the outset
- evaluate for learning and for judgement; an 'improvement' orientation (how to get better next time) as well as a 'dials' orientation (marks out of ten) that together ensures that regardless of what happened there is a chance that whatever has been learned will help it to be better the next time around.

Unfortunately, evaluation is one of the weaker aspects of EBD to date, and it has to be said that it has not really attracted the level of attention that it merits. Indeed, what often passes as evaluation may be little more than a cursory retrospective. Even more usually, there is no evaluation at all, and therefore no evidence base that others can learn from. In the overall scheme of things, the Lambeth, Lewisham and Southwark project described earlier[2] is therefore impressive because it did seek to look back in order to identify what had changed and how participants thought and felt about their co-design experiences. Unfortunately, however, there was no outcomes evaluation in terms of whether services themselves – and particularly patients' experiences of those services – had improved as a result of the project.

Readers may be aware of the distinction between formative and summative evaluation which needs to be introduced into our discussion at this point.

Formative evaluation

This is a form of 'action research' whereby the results of the evaluation are constantly fed back to inform the ongoing development and improvement of the project or programme, making it integral to the intervention and implementation itself. We call this evaluation for learning ('how can we learn and get better as we go?'). Action research is now quite widespread in UK health but, nevertheless, is still viewed in many circles as less weighty and essential than summative evaluations and not 'good science' because one is intervening in and influencing the situation one is purportedly trying to measure. Battles between both camps are often bloody and bitter, with the formative evaluators, for their part, retaliating by asking what is the point of a summative evaluation that reports long after crucial decisions have been taken (say to spread or curtail a project), or after all the 'damage' has been done, and which had it been fed in to the process might have saved the project from failure or improved its chance of success.[3,4]

Summative evaluation

This second type, as exemplified by the Lambeth study, is retrospective, after the event evaluation (*ex ante* or *ex post*) that seeks to ascertain whether and to what extent the programme or project was implemented as intended and the desired/anticipated results achieved. The purpose is to ensure accountability and value for money, with the results of the evaluation informing any future planning decisions, policy and resource allocation. We call this evaluation for judgement ('how did we do?'). Carrying out this type of summative – literally 'summing up' – evaluation has become almost obligatory in the public sector where there has been growing demand in recent years for greater accountability and value for money,[5] although doubts remain as to what happens to the evidence from such evaluations and, coming as late as it does, whether it even alters the course of events.[3,4,6]

Up until now, whatever evaluation there has been of EBD or similar design, interventions have been mainly of the summative kind, geared to finding out whether and to what extent patient experience or satisfaction with the service (*see* below) have improved as a result of the intervention. This is a pity because, arguably, the spirit of collaboration that imbues EBD and interactive design with its distinctive quality is more suited to the notion of formative – and informative – developmental evaluation, or better still a combination of both.

Formative evaluation of EBD

Formative evaluation of the pilot

Using the pilot (*see* Chapter 9) as an example of how this kind of evaluation may be done in an EBD context, Box E summarises our core team's reflections – captured formatively during the pilot – on how we might 'do it better' next time. These reflections address specific elements of the EBD process (for example, the co-design events, the use of film) rather than the process as a whole, and were captured throughout the pilot during discussions at core project team meetings and after key events. These reflections were then used to make any necessary course adjustments and to 'design out' any problems reagarding future actions and activities. Further detailed advice and suggestions for those interested in implementing and evaluating EBD in their own organisations are available from the NHSi's website: www. institute.nhs.uk/quality_and_value/introduction/experience_based_design.html.

Box E: Reflections: how to do it better next time?

> *Reflection – true reflection – leads to action. (Paolo Freire)*

Here we present some of the reflections of the core group charged with introducing the EBD process to the head and neck service that participated in the pilot study described in Chapter 9. These brief reflections take the form of 10 specific questions that practitioners or service improvement specialists may find helpful once they have familiarised themselves with the EBD process used in the pilot study.

1 **Why is it necessary to commit so much time and effort to capturing staff views (when it is supposed to be patient experiences we are after)?**

- EBD is a form of OD and hence the same rules of 'good change' apply, namely that 'authorship equals ownership' or that a 'change imposed is a change opposed'.

- The experience of giving the service is as relevant and important to design as the experience of receiving it; the design process needs to take account of both, and it is the bringing together of these two perspectives in the same room that gives EBD its unique energy and insight.
- Working with staff from the outset helps them get attuned to EBD and the meaning of 'experience' and the role they can play in shaping it. At the same time one is also building the change relationship and creating the necessary readiness for change for the design process to begin.
- Staff have an important role to play in the early stages of an EBD project such as identifying informants, familiarising the researchers and designers with the service and the context, advising on prototypes of new tools and methods, and identifying possible patients and carer volunteers for the co-design group.
- Without this initial period of intense interaction with staff there would have been insufficient levels of goodwill and trust to initiate and sustain the EBD process.

2 **How could we have improved the first co-design event?**

- Getting people active sooner with fewer presentations and more tasks.
- More live storytelling (first hand) to 'reawaken' experiences as well as use of filmed interviews (second hand). One radical proposal would be to ask patients and staff to tell their stories 'live', and to pull out touch points and design principles as they go. This may be possible for co-design groups that have some experience of working together but less so for newcomers to EBD.
- Pairs and trios rather than larger group-work to encourage personal responsibility (and reduce group-think and staff-talk).
- Make greater use of the experience and emotion maps from the staff feedback event.

3 **How can we make the 'voices' of the various participants more equal?**

- Encourage and facilitate co-presentations from a patient and staff member.
- Pre-briefing of staff to make them aware of the need to bring patients in.
- Clearly focus participation in the EBD process around the common, shared goals of improving services and the patient experience.

4 **How can we maximise the potential value of all the rich in-depth interview data we collected as part of the EBD process?**

- We used this data to (a) prepare the detailed feedback to the staff (via the clinical director) and (b) generate the key stages in the patient journey, the touch points and emotions that went into the overall 'patient experience' map used at the patient feedback day.
- The co-design event could have gone further by explicitly comparing the touch points as identified by (a) staff and (b) patients, perhaps using the four touch-point scenarios described on p. 146 in Chapter 9. This might have been a good way of starting the co-design event.

5 **Are there more effective ways of identifying and developing actions around touch points and design principles?**

- Generally speaking we have found that patients and staff find touch points an easier concept to grasp than design principles. Nonetheless the latter have played a key role in steering the process towards implementation and closure.

6 **Are we using the films of the patients and staff in a way that maximises their potential contribution?**

- Next time we would make sure that patients also see the film of the staff event to stimulate dialogue and gain an understanding of their approach and 'take' on the issues in advance.
- The films could be edited down into targeted clips, tailored to specific touch points and the respective individual co-design groups (for example, at the PEG or radiotherapy 'experience').
- Staff and patients could be given a personal copy of the film to take away and watch again if they so wished as it may be too much to take in all at once at first viewing.

7 **What should be the role (if any) of external researchers?**

- Many of those involved with the process were in favour of retaining the research(er) component. The senior surgeon on the advisory group was concerned that an EBD process that jumped the research stage would not capture the key issues and challenges (or touch points) in as effective a way as the researchers had done.
- Patients and carers might prefer to raise and talk through issues with a non-partisan third party without staff being present; this third party might be someone from a Patient & Public Involvement Group and/or at times might even be another patient (as is in fact now starting to happen at the pilot site).
- Through their observational role the researchers had been able to see things that staff (and even sometimes patients) had not been aware of or able to see (certainly the weighing scales, red line and language in the consultation would not have been identified).
- Although not all EBD projects will have the resources for external researchers our recommendation would be to include them if possible, recognising that it is not just about data gathering or analysis (which internal staff could learn to do for themselves over time) but the fact that the very presence of a third party will affect the dynamics of the process.

8 **How important is it to span and take account of the whole patient journey in an EBD process?**

- In this case study we think we focused too much on the head and neck outpatient clinic at the expense of other key stages of the patient journey (for example, radiotherapy or primary care). This naturally resulted in priorities for improvement focusing on the clinic rather than the other areas (although later activities have included one patient acting as a 'mystery shopper' at a patient orientation visit at the radiotherapy centre).

- One possibility would be to break the whole patient journey down into discrete stages for different co-design events.

9 How sustainable is the process and resulting improvements?

- In discussion with the advisory group we identified three main potential drivers for sustainability: (a) patients and carers carrying on with the work for themselves; (b) staff feeling sufficiently energised by the process and the mobilising narratives that had been heard and seen; and (c) 'old-fashioned' management systems.
- We would suggest that all three of the above drivers probably need to be active if improvements identified by an EBD process are to be first implemented and then sustained. However, it was not until near the end of our case study that we came to realise that the EBD actions had not been, for example, integrated into the management of the surgical directorate.
- We believe that implementation does need to occur as part of an extracurricular process (so as to allow all the special things we observed – energy, passion, momentum – to manifest themselves) but that sustainability and spread do require the judicious use of the mainstream management system and all the skills and resources available to it.
- In this case study we took action by firming up the list of changes that each of the six groups had signed up to; this became the core group's checklist for monitoring (against agreed deadlines) what had or hadn't been done by the time of the second co-design event.

10 Is there a need to look for alternative models of EBD?

- One way of getting the process more internally owned and self-managing would be for the researchers to drop out and be replaced by a process in which 'pairs' or trios of clinicians/staff and patients/carers form around the care process (this could be thought of as a joint action learning project where the parties form an improvement 'compact' to go through various design stages together).
- There may be advantages in having researchers and designers shift their roles from central project management to being 'on-call' to provide assistance and support to individuals and groups as required.

Other methods and tools of formative evaluation

There are other formative evaluation methods not used in our work that might provide alternative or complementary approaches to what we have described. For example, although not strictly from the world of design, the 'dialogical, story-based evaluation tool' developed by Dart and Davies[7] might be useful not least because of the firm roots that it has in the narrative, storytelling approaches to design described earlier (*see* Chapters 6 and 8), which mostly make EBD what it is. It is called the 'most significant change' (MSC) technique, and was originally developed, in fact is still widely used, by international organisations working in the field of rural development and improvement. Its primary purpose, as a formative intervention, is to facilitate programme improvement by focusing the direction of work towards explicitly valued directions and away from less valued directions.

The MSC involves the ongoing collection and participatory interpretation of 'stories' about change or improvement arising from the programme, rather than (or, if one prefers, in tandem with) predetermined indicators. A similar approach (albeit related to strategic change in a single organisation) is that of dialogue-based planning, a tool recently developed and employed in healthcare by McKinsey Consulting.[8] In the case of EBD, such collection, interpretation and evaluation activities would become integral to the co-design process itself, include patient, staff and user stories, and most likely centre on touch points and/or critical incidents (the MSC's authors themselves point to the similarities with critical incident reporting and results mapping). The stories, then, are a form of ongoing self-evaluation, the advantages of this approach being, first, that it creates an ongoing process of learning and reflection, and therefore arguably a more successful improvement process overall; second, that it brings the evaluation process into the (ongoing) present, causing people to confront any pressing issues and problems in the here and now rather than leaving them until it is possibly too late; and third, stimulating an interactive, subjective and inter-subjective process that is the best and possibly only way of getting at experience. After all, how else can we discover whether a person's experience has improved other than by asking them and giving them the opportunity to say whether it has or not? By its very nature, experience needs to be evaluated emically from the actor's point of view not etically or externally, as would more likely occur in a summative evaluation.

In the MSC, the stories are collected with the help of a simple question: 'During the last month [could be more could be less], in your opinion, what was the most significant change that took place in this domain of the programme?' As part of the formative design process, those involved in the case study site might therefore talk and discuss the significance of any changes that had taken place in such touch-point domains as the post-operative ward, the clinic, the PEG, and radiotherapy (*see* Chapter 9), naturalistically through stories and anecdotes rather than any objective or detached kind of process. In line with the method, they would also be encouraged to report why they consider a particular change to be the most significant one, the implication being that it is significant either because it is moving in the right direction towards the valued direction or away from it. Thus armed with the 'what' and the 'why' of change, participants would be able to plan what action needs to be taken to consolidate the gain, continue to move the changes in the positive direction, or to put the intervention back on track.

Stories are a valuable part of the MSC for several reasons: they encourage non-evaluation experts to participate, indeed to become the evaluators themselves and own and conduct what is essentially an internal self-evaluation (with external monitoring if deemed necessary); they are likely to be remembered as a complex whole; and they can help keep the dialogue based on concrete issues and outcomes rather than abstract indicators. The filtering, flow and feedback of 'key stories' through and across different lines of authority in the organisation can also assist in the accumulation and spread of learning, and the derivation of general design rules for application to other services (*see* Chapter 7), and can at any time be used to check for accuracy and veracity by visiting the area in question and comparing the rhetoric with the action. Stories can also be gathered together into a video or book compendium, which can stand as a record and source reference for various kinds of summative qualitative and quantitative analysis, for processes such as round-table and steering group meetings, and as a monitor for the sustainability of the improvements.

Summative evaluation of EBD

If the aim of EBD is to improve users' experience of the services they receive, then clearly this is where any evaluation needs to be directed. There are numerous survey tools that at least purport to measure patient experience in healthcare, [9–15] most of which can be used diagnostically (*see* Chapter 8) or evaluatively. As will be clear from the following, the differences between this type of tool and the previous one are quite marked, summative evaluation and survey tools being mostly 'etic' (designed, administered and analysed by non-users of the service, including the choice of things that supposedly make up user experience), quantitative/numbers-based rather than qualitative/stories-based, and 'still' snapshots (mainly, although not always, taken at the end) rather than moving processes. One further difference is that summative tools do not tend to make any strong distinction between 'perceptions/attitudes' and 'experiences' (and similarly between 'satisfaction' and a 'good experience'), the most probable reason being that the latter are difficult, if not impossible, to capture on a rating scale and, despite the researcher's good intentions, often end up bearing a closer resemblance to the former.

Summative evaluations may involve either survey or interview methods or a combination of both.

Summative evaluation using surveys

NHS satisfaction and experience surveys

One of the more interesting tools is the Trent Health Authority 'Patient Centrometer'.[9] The 'Patient Centrometer' is a hybrid tool (summative and formative) developed in the Trent region of England that is intended to gather patients' feedback based on their experiences. A service evaluation team visits ward areas at pre-arranged times and talks to patients using the questionnaire to structure the conversation. This information is synthesised and can then be fed back to the ward, or organisation or relevant strategic health authority, and a plan for action/change is devised. Local service improvement teams can then help the ward team make the changes that are needed. Other interesting activities to augment the process include working with patients who have dementia and using collage – images selected or described by patients – to create a picture which is then looked at by psychologists who try to define some of the key messages. Patient workshop settings are also used to help

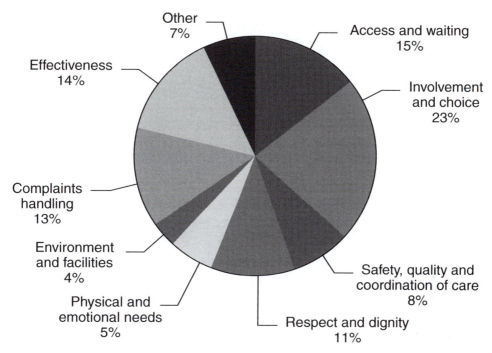

Figure 10.1   Breakdown of NHS complaints received by the Healthcare Commission (for Trusts in England). *Source:* Healthcare Commission.[15]

identify what patients feel 'sad, mad or glad' about, which they embellish with a particular story.

Alternatively, patient complaints are sometimes used as a proxy for 'patient experience'. In England, the Healthcare Commission is responsible for reviewing complaints about the NHS that have not been resolved locally. These are called 'second stage complaints'. From July 2004 to May 2005, the Commission received more than 7,000 complaints, purportedly covering all aspects of 'people's experiences of healthcare' (*see* Figure 10.1) and suggested that lessons about designing systems from the point of view of the user can also emerge from people's complaints about healthcare in the NHS.[16]

We are aware that readers will already have picked up on the reservations and concerns we have about some of the summative and survey evaluation tools currently in use, all of which prompts us to urge caution in their use, at least in an EBD setting. As we have said, a lot of what reviewing complaints and other of the approaches and surveys referenced focus upon is attitudes rather than experience, which recalls our earlier point that a survey may be able to get at the former but it will have greater difficulty with the latter. In some cases such tools are indistinguishable from patient satisfaction surveys, and even use 'satisfaction' and 'experience' interchangeably in their writing. And yet we know that though clearly related (i.e. a bad experience will make you dissatisfied) there is a difference. Kale, for example, points out that 'the difference between satisfaction and quality is not merely semantic. Satisfaction relates to a single transaction and is consumption-specific',[17] and goes on to point out that 'services research is replete with incidences where people are satisfied with a particular services provider but did not perceive the service firm to be of high quality.' He suggests that:

> customer satisfaction surveys seldom provide any insights into customer loyalty . . . Instead of pouring money into the coffers of well-meaning but conceptually unenlightened market research firms to obtain customer satisfaction ratings, you will be better off investing in sound instruments that track service quality.

The practical implication here is that a project to improve user satisfaction may end up being quite different from one that seeks to improve the quality of user experience.

Another reservation we have is that while survey tools may be strong in areas such as privacy and dignity, there remains a gaping hole in the area of emotional experience. Users are simply not asked 'how did it feel?', or how those feelings or the mix of them may have changed as they went through the various stages of their (emotional) rollercoaster journey. In this respect one senses that none of them have really moved far from the traditional scientific approach of mapping the experience 'etically' using the (cool, detached) framework of the expert outsider, or have seriously tried to discover how it looks and feels from the inside 'emic' point of view of the patient or carer.

As a further illustration, Sandoval and colleagues[18] used a survey tool to assess factors which influence cancer patients' perceptions of the quality of their care. Their study explained between 25 and 34% of the variance of the overall perception of quality by means of four predictors: information about follow-up care after completing treatment; knew next step in care; knew who to go to with questions; and providers were aware of test results. The authors suggest that 'practitioners' improvement efforts might be constructively focused on the four predictors mentioned'. For us, all this serves to do is to highlight the dangers of relying on questionnaire surveys. Recall the patients in the case study who – with regard to the second predictors above – made quite clear that had they known the next step was radiotherapy treatment (and all that entailed) they would have 'laid down' (*see* page 151). To paraphrase Van Maanen, satisfaction surveys are all too often an 'armchair mode of investigation' carried out at a safe distance from the action, which is precisely what makes relying upon them so dangerous. Finally, and just as importantly, many of these approaches and surveys are, unlike EBD, not part of a larger OD process and as Davies and Cleary[19] point out:

> . . . surveys themselves do not indicate what needs to be done to improve any situation. Further commitment and ingenuity are needed to understand shortcomings in an organisation and develop solutions.

Summative survey-type measures from the design sciences

There are already a number of tools in the design field itself that have the potential for adaptation or adoption in EBD interventions and evaluations within healthcare. Take Robert Rubinoff's 'quick and dirty' methodology for 'objectively' quantifying the user experience,[20] which although designed to evaluate websites could be used for high-level or overview evaluations in a service setting like healthcare. He says that the user experience is primarily made up of four interdependent elements (note also how he brings physical and experience design together as did Hester in Manteo – *see* Chapter 8):

- branding: visual impact, signage, media, a product or service that delivers what it says 'on the side of the can', and a branding that is fitting for the nature of the service or product
- functionality: users receive timely responses, messages and instructions are clearly communicated, the service is efficient, and delivers what it is supposed to deliver
- usability: interaction between service and user is sufficiently 'user-friendly' to prevent errors, and accomplish their goals, and
- content: clarity and easy navigation, content is up-to-date, accurate, and appropriate to user needs and organisational goals.

Branding

Statement	Scale	Score
Statement 1	1 - 20	15
Statement 2	1 - 20	11
Statement 3	1 - 20	8
Statement 4	1 - 20	18
Statement 5	1 - 20	6
Branding TOTAL:		**58 of 100**

Functionality

Statement	Scale	Score
Statement 1	1 - 20	11
Statement 2	1 - 20	6
Statement 3	1 - 20	8
Statement 4	1 - 20	2
Statement 5	1 - 20	5
Functionality TOTAL:		**32 of 100**

Usability

Statement	Scale	Score
Statement 1	1 - 20	4
Statement 2	1 - 20	10
Statement 3	1 - 20	18
Statement 4	1 - 20	7
Statement 5	1 - 20	6
Usability TOTAL:		**45 of 100**

Content

Statement	Scale	Score
Statement 1	1 - 20	7
Statement 2	1 - 20	9
Statement 3	1 - 20	3
Statement 4	1 - 20	10
Statement 5	1 - 20	8
Content TOTAL:		**37 of 100**

Make sure that the sum of the maximum possible scores for the entire element equals 100. This results in a true percentage for each of the elements.

In the end, you'll have 4 separate scores (1 score for each of the four elements) that you can then plot using a spreadsheet or graphing program.

Figure 10.2 Customer experience measure. *Source:* Rubinoff.[19]

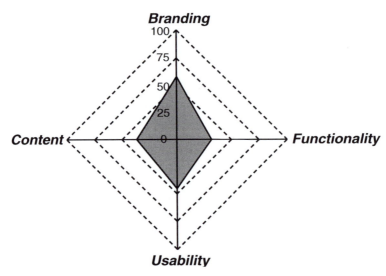

Figure 10.3 Spider chart. *Source:* Rubinoff.[19]

> *Independently, none of these factors makes for positive user experience; however, taken together, these factors constitute the main ingredients for . . . success. Each is accompanied by five statements that users rate on a scale of 1–20, for example 'the site provides visitors with an engaging and memorable experience'. (see Figure 10.2)*

Finally, once the analysis has been completed and values arrived at for each of the statements or parameters, the final task is to put this data into a clear, communicative format, such as a spider chart (*see* Figure 10.3).

There are numerous design consultancies specialising in similar kinds of methods, more often than not used to improve the 'usability' of websites (as in the case of Rubinoff's tool described above), but including broader evaluation services such as developing user profiles, identifying user needs, analysing task needs, conducting exploratory and participatory design studies, and conducting product usability tests. For readers who want to know more, a good sample of these can be found by Googling 'usability reviews and testing', a search that will throw up, for example, *Discovering User Needs: Field Techniques You Can Use*.[21] More specifically still, a Google search of 'measuring customer experience' retrieves 199 hits and a plethora of 'customer experience' survey tools and metrics grouped under headings like 'customer relationship management,' 'customer relationship metrics', 'customer experience management' or 'customer experience research', and all promising 'a set of measures and indices that capture the critical drivers for customer experience [going] beyond traditional and unilateral customer satisfaction studies'. Interestingly, only one of these is directly related to a healthcare setting,[22] although this is not really a problem because many of these applications could easily be adapted for use in this area.

Evaluation of user experiences in the design field usually involves the initial identification of a number of key dimensions (seven or thereabouts) to measure. As an example, Publicom[23] is fairly typical in this regard: expounding on arguments from Joe Pine and Jim Gilmore's bestseller *The Experience Economy*, collaborators from Publicom (a services marketing consultancy) and Michigan State University were intrigued by the authors' indications of movement out of the service economy toward what they called the experience economy, and began to carry out their own work to identify and measure the components of an experience. The seven dimensions of the consumer's buying experience identified in the study are:

- driving benefit: understanding how to use a product or service, as well as its consistency, benefit and value
- accessibility: product or service must be readily available or easy to acquire
- convenience: the entire shopping process should be fast; products or services easy to locate
- incentives: offering incentives increase the chance of buying the featured product or service
- utility: practicality is important; there should be no surprises surrounding a product or service; safety is a major concern
- brand trust: satisfaction with a store or product or service is critical, and
- sales environment: surroundings should be entertaining, stimulating, educational.

Jeffrey Beck, one of the study's researchers, summed up what he thought their contribution had been:

> *An experience, while a distinct economic offering, had gone largely unrecognized, unstudied and unmeasured. Our study is significant because it's the first step in identifying and measuring the underlying dimensions that are important in a customer experience.*[23]

While most of the items on their list will by now be very familiar to readers (the user-experience honeycomb in Chapter 2 and Figure 2.4 is very similar), they are worth repeating because, in our view, they could quite easily form the basis of a healthcare evaluation tool (survey or interview) for assessing some key aspects of the patient experience.

Why the NHS needs to revisit its 'experience' survey measures

The Department of Health's own public service agreement aims and objectives includes specific reference to 'patient experience'. As we discussed in Chapter 1, one of the 12 objectives agreed between the Department of Health and the Treasury in 2002 was to improve service standards by enhancing 'accountability to patients and the public and [securing] sustained national improvements in *patient experience* [our emphasis] as measured by independently validated national surveys'.[24] This target was amended in 2004 to read 'secure sustained annual national improvements in NHS patient experience by 2008, as measured by independently validated surveys, ensuring that individuals are fully involved in decisions about their health care, including choice of provider'. In 2004 the Department reported that:

> *Trusts are continuing to gather the views of patients through the national patient survey programme . . . designed not only to provide patient feedback at a national level, but also to provide local feedback to be used by individual Trusts for quality improvement.*24

Responsibility for patient 'surveys' (their term) was taken over by the Healthcare Commission in April 2004, which carried out five national surveys that year asking patients across England about their 'experiences of mental health, inpatient, ambulance, paediatric and primary care services'. As the Healthcare Commission's website states:

> the surveys in the NHS patient survey programme provide the data for calculating the scores on the experiences of patients used to monitor the Department of Health's public service agreement target on the experiences of patients.[25]

Whilst it is encouraging to see the two major planks of EBD, participation and experience, figuring so prominently in Department of Health thinking, it still leaves the question: do surveys such as they are using really get at experience, and is there a danger that they are confusing this, yet again, with attitudes, opinions and satisfaction? Even the Department itself would appear to have some reservations. For instance, in its Autumn Performance Report for 2005, it is noted that:

> The Department [of Health] designed the methodology used to measure improvements in the patient experience in collaboration with the Healthcare Commission. Since the PSA technical note was first published, the Healthcare Commission has proposed a change to the methodology. DH is working with the Healthcare Commission to review the proposed change and other aspects of the methodology . . .[26]

Changes were indeed made but the survey approach was retained, in fact was never questioned nor, it would seem, alternatives considered. Thus in May 2006 the Healthcare Commission continued to suggest that 'the [national patient] survey captures the *experiences* of over 80,000 adult patients' [our emphasis].[27] The survey was carried out by the Picker Institute on behalf of the Commission and their joint website (www.nhssurveys.org) carries the strapline 'focus on patients' experiences'. We are not arguing that such surveys are without value (although as already noted they cannot in themselves lead to improvement – there is a disconnect between evaluation of this nature and the improvement process[19]), simply that they may not be measuring experiences. Coulter from the Picker Institute argues that 'patients' surveys should ask about real experiences of medical care'[28] but what is the point of asking if they don't actually provide any sensible answers? We leave readers to judge for themselves whether surveys really do get at, or, even more ambitious still, can measure, 'experience'. Can a survey really measure the experience of love or loss, joy or pain? Can they ever represent it from the actor's point of view and in their own words when the questions are structured around someone else's language and conceptual framework? Can a – by definition – qualitative phenomenon like experience ever hope to be captured quantitatively in numbers and rating scales?

Our view in summary is, first, that other methods and approaches to evaluation such as those described elsewhere in this chapter need to be considered. Second, surveys should only be used to measure what they can actually measure, for example the more objective and technical aspects of quality:

> Well designed questionnaires for patients could contribute usefully to an assessment of both the technical competence and interpersonal skills of doctors. If these surveys are to play a role in quality improvement, they should provide clear factual results that prompt follow-up actions.[28]

Third, they should not claim to be measuring one thing, like experience, when they are actually measuring something else, like satisfaction – for example, a general practice assessment survey comprising nine so-called 'experience domains' only asks about satisfaction: access to practice; satisfaction with receptionists; satisfaction with continuity of care; satisfaction with communication; satisfaction with interpersonal care; trust in general practitioner; general practitioner's knowledge; satisfaction with practice nursing; and satisfaction with technical care (cited Rao and colleagues[29]). So we know that a patient was dissatisfied with the receptionist, but do we really know anything about her experience of that interaction and how it was felt, and what particular part of it prompted this negative response? And do we have any 'valid information' at all (to use the OD phrase) with which to begin to make it a better experience for her, and no doubt the receptionist, the next time around? The answer must be a no to both questions.

And, fourth, steps could be taken now to diversify methodologies and effect improvements to existing tools. For example, Coulter proposes that instead of asking patients to rate their care using general evaluation categories (such as excellent, very good, good, fair, poor), it might be better to ask them to report in detail on their experiences of clinical care during a particular consultation (for instance, 'Were you given information about any side effects of your medicine?'), a specific episode of care ('Were you given a plan to help you manage your diabetes at home?'), or over a specified period ('Have you had your blood pressure checked in the past 12 months?').[28] These types of question are designed to elicit reports on what actually occurred, rather than the patient's evaluation of what occurred, and they produce more reliable results.

Summative evaluation using interviews

Here we present the findings from the EBD pilot described in Chapter 9 to illustrate how interviews may be used in place of surveys to provide the summative component of an EBD evaluation. The findings are based on in-depth interviews with staff and patients who participated in the pilot. Interviews were typically of one to two hours duration and were tape-recorded and transcribed. Box F shows the type of questions covered and the range of issues discussed. These were very much a collaborative effort involving both the core project team and advisory group, our belief being that the evaluation should address questions considered relevant by those directly involved and to which they were genuinely seeking answers. This is very different to most summative methods which tend to allow only very limited user participation in question formulation:

Box F: Evaluation interviews

Tell us the story of your involvement in this project; how did you come to be involved?

  Looking back over your involvement since then:

- How would you describe what you and others have been doing to someone who did not know about it?
- What has it felt like to be involved?

- [STAFF ONLY] How has this project been different to other improve-
  ment projects you have been involved with in the past (or are involved
  with right now)? Why has it been different?
- Tell us one good or successful story from the process . . . and one not so
  good, or a disappointment.
- What improvements have you seen in the head and neck service? Can
  you give examples/anecdotes? Do you think they will last?
- Do you think the head and neck service is more efficient now? Why?
  Examples?
- Do you think the head and neck service is any safer now? Why?
  Examples?
- What has improved in terms of the patient experience of the head and
  neck service?
- What have been the most important parts of the project/process from
  your perspective? Why were they important?
- Anything you think should have been done differently as part of the
  process (i.e. to make it better)?
- How have you found working closely with patients/staff? Has working
  closely with patients/staff made a difference? Was it as you expected it
  to be?
- Would you recommend this as something for other staff/patients to get
  involved with? Can you give reasons as to why you might recommend
  it to other patients/staff as an activity to participate in?
- Are there any aspects to the head and neck service that you still think
  need to be improved urgently?
- What do you think will happen now? Will the work continue? In what
  way/form?

The findings of the interviews are organised here into four sub-sections:

1 What specific improvements in (a) performance, (b) safety and (c) patient
   experience were implemented as a result of the EBD pilot?
2 What did patients and staff perceive as the central characteristics of the EBD
   approach?
3 What did participants identify as the 'must do's' or key success factors of an
   EBD approach?
4 What can the pilot tell us about the likely spread and sustainability of
   improvements brought about by an EBD approach?

1 What specific improvements in (a) performance, (b) safety and (c) patient experience were implemented as a result of the EBD pilot?

In short, this is the traditional summative 'did EBD work?' question. To begin to
answer it, during the course of the pilot the local service improvement facilitator
co-ordinating the project maintained a register of all the specific improvements
made to the head and neck cancer service as a direct result of the project. This list

provided a breakdown of the 'experiences that need improving' as identified by patients and/or staff and the subsequent actions taken by the six co-design groups (*see* Table 9.1) to improve these experiences over the course of the pilot.

In this case 43 specific improvements were recorded and many of these were brought about by more than one action taken by patient and/or staff. For example, one improvement – to enable patients to fully understand the nature of the 'radiotherapy planning' appointment – has been addressed by three separate actions. In total across the 43 improvements, 70 actions were implemented. Many seemingly minor changes (for example, moving the weighing scales) which were found to be impacting in a significant and negative way on patient experiences were actioned almost immediately; other issues (for example, levels of staff training on the post-operative ward) are still being addressed through longer-term solutions.

Overall comments

Before describing the specific improvements identified by interviewees, a number of general observations as to the impact and merits of EBD were made. Participants in the pilot were overwhelmingly positive in their views as to its value:

> *I think it is definitely worth it. I think it is invaluable, even if it is just a one-off but to have sessions where patients can feed back to you about your service, I think is the only way that you are going to be able to build your service and move forward.* (support staff)

> *It definitely has changed the service and interaction with the patients, the way that we're interacting, it's absolutely brilliant, and I would recommend it for other groups to work in this way, but staff need the support. I also think some members of staff will be able to work in this way better than others.* (nurse)

> *I don't know how it could have been made better. I thought the whole project was first class.* (patient)

> *I think that everybody's been quite enthusiastic about the whole thing and they're still talking about it because the whole project's still being shown in various other meetings with the film, so they have been very positive about the whole thing . . . it's very positive.* (surgeon)

More specifically, the EBD project was credited by participants as having enabled staff to make improvements to the head and neck service that had been long planned but which had previously not been implemented:

> *I know that one member of staff has battled away to try and get another specialist to do stuff, and battled away with ward managers to try and get them to do stuff, and they've not been successful. But this [EBD] has taken it away from any one staff member trying to get another one to do the right thing because now we've got a collective group if you like of staff and patients and certainly people who will say, 'this is important that we do something about it'. And they're forcing the hand of the people who have not come up with the goods previously really; I think it's had that sort of effect.* (support staff)

> *Certainly all the staff I've met have impressed me with their enthusiasm for the project, and enthusiasm for improvement. It's almost as though there's been*

some sort of injection into the staff. I think it's something that was perhaps waiting to happen, and they needed a catalyst I think. (patient)

Staff also commented that the pilot had helped them to recognise that what had been thought of previously as marginal parts of service (or relatively trivial aspects) are, in fact, central to the overall patient experience of the service, and the work had therefore given them a much greater understanding of the whole patient journey:

> *for members of staff to see what the patients' experience of radiotherapy is and the mask because they just don't understand or they haven't had an under-standing; they know people go for radiotherapy but what does that involve? And when they actually see the mask [on film], I think they get a much better idea, definitely.* (nursing staff)

> *like the PEG group – part of their experience of delivering care is that they feel PEG isn't important in the whole scheme of things; they feel a bit marginalised, an add on, an afterthought . . . I think [EBD] has gone a little way to having them as much part of parcel of it . . . It's definitely given them an opportunity to flag up their area and as the patients are saying 'it's an important part of my experience' that naturally puts them a bit more central. If other staff are hear-ing that too, then those staff are realising that PEG is much more central to the experience than they've probably given it credit for previously.* (support staff)

> *and I think what this has highlighted, listening to them [the patients] speak-ing is it's the tiny, tiny, little things that seem to have the biggest impact . . . it's their day-to-day living really where we're having the most impact and it's how they actually rearrange their routines and their lifestyle, and it's the tiny little things that they always come out and say.* (nursing staff)

Specific improvements

We argued earlier (*see* Figure 1.1 and Chapter 2) that there are three basic things that healthcare improvement efforts should be looking for and taken as a com-plete bundle or package: performance, engineering and aesthetics. To illustrate the all too common trade-offs between one or more of these components, the EBD pilot described in Chapter 9 uncovered a number of potential instances of what might be termed 'great process (i.e. performance) but terrible experience (i.e. aesthetics)':

> *this is very much about recognising that we're improving processes and trying to get people to move fast but absolutely not wanting to forget the patients' experience in that. Recognising that good processes aren't necessarily a good experience . . .* (support staff)

> *Maybe the patients don't feel it, maybe it's the staff that are feeling it, because I get very frustrated when patients are rushed through, and I think some of it is to do with the wait and obviously the quicker we treat patients, the better chance we have of curing them. There is obviously that side, but you have got to put some of the quality stuff in there, so the time spent with patients before their treatment, explaining what is going to happen, which we do a lot of, if we're not careful, that gets really hurried along and the patients get very con-fused, and they don't have the time to process what is going on, and I know*

that is a national problem . . . So we just need to keep a check on that. It would be really, really sad if after all this the quality of what we do comes down. (therapist)

Below we provide examples of improvements made in terms of each of these components which combined – rather than conflicted – with the other two components. However, as one participant commented:

this [the pilot] is about patients and staff experience and yes, hopefully, you get some real positive outcomes in terms of efficiency and effectiveness. But I don't think that's the main emphasis here, I think the main emphasis is about improving the experiences. (support staff)

(a) Performance

Two specific 'performance' improvements were identified. One experience that needed improving originated initially from a staff perception that 'the seating [in the outpatient clinic] is cramped and there are too many people waiting', later supplemented by patient comments about their initial reactions to seeing the clinic for the first time. In part response to this, patients and staff came into the clinic one morning and rearranged the physical layout of the clinic (*see* comments under (c) below). However, other actions taken were much more focused on improving efficiency via the flow of patients through the fortnightly clinic in order to reduce waiting times for appointments and over-crowding:

they're moving long-term follow up patients out of the clinic as they're seeing them so that's an ongoing process . . . they are more efficient in that they are thinking more acutely about how they're using their resources and their time, and their clinic space and their clinic slots. (support staff)

with the clinic that's been good in that we're moving some of the appointments, so patients are going on to the regular clinic, so I think that's good because that will free up time and give more time for patients in the combined clinic . . . it will be more efficient in terms of the organising and management of the service as a result obviously from the patients' experiences . . . we have four or five different options in reorganising the clinic rooms so I feel that will be more effective, too. (nursing staff)

This example of a performance improvement resulting from an EBD touch point highlights how a focus on experience can be a means of identifying topics or issues which are then best addressed by other improvement techniques (for example, Lean process redesign) which are designed to directly impact on performance. Furthermore, whilst many of the documented 43 improvements have been planned and implemented by patients and staff working closely together in one of the six co-design groups, the rescheduling of the clinic appointments is an example of a staff-led initiative to improve both their own and their patients' experiences which has a knock-on effect in terms of performance:

things like re-pacing the appointments means that the waiting room is less stuffed so when a patient walks around the corner it doesn't look so full of people, people standing and waiting for seats and things. And the patients couldn't have done that but the fact that they pointed out the experience of the clinic has prompted staff to think 'hold on a minute; we've been putting these appointments in these couple of hours and getting people in but what's the impact of this?' We're now realising what that's actually doing to people and how they're experiencing that. I don't think the patients could have done anything about that; that had to be a staff action. (support staff)

In this pilot perhaps the best example of EBD and Lean 'coming together' was when – as a result of the patient stories about their experiences on the post-surgical ward – Lean techniques were employed to make changes to the ward environment to improve working conditions for staff, with the knock-on effect of improving patient experiences too.

(b) Engineering (being safe and feeling safe)

Four specific 'safety' improvements were identified. To take one example, patient interviews had highlighted that some patients did not feel safe on the post-surgical ward, an issue not necessarily obvious to non-ward based clinical staff (*see* second quotation):

I think where patients have really contributed to the ward staff is by telling their stories of how safe or unsafe they felt in the ward situation. And examples they were giving were things like the hand washing; 'I'm not sure that everybody washes their hands and particularly visitors', and 'my tube came out on Saturday morning and nobody knew how to put it back in' and that has made staff have to sit up and think about the skill sets amongst the staff and ways in which they can try and make sure that seven days a week there's somebody who knows how to. (support staff)

it's interesting to hear what people actually on the receiving end tell us . . . it's interesting to hear people's views when they are being a patient on the ward because we see them for minutes on a daily basis but they're there 24 hours a day, so it's the other hours that we weren't there that we didn't know what's going on. (surgeon)

As a further example of the actions that have resulted subsequently, three specific changes have been implemented – or are now underway – to address the specific issue of reinserting the stomagastric feeding tube: a training needs analysis of all staff on the ward; the modification of a tracheotomy booklet from another hospital for use as revision for existing staff and as part of the induction of new staff; and the development of an integrated care pathway for laryngectomy patients.

As with the 'performance' example above, it is important to highlight the way in which EBD and other improvement activities – in this case a concurrent hospital-wide patient safety initiative – can combine to good effect; EBD provides a different perspective on safety issues that can then be addressed through the most appropriate mechanism available. It is therefore about more than just experience improvement.

(c) Aesthetics (patient and staff experience)

The vast majority of the improvements made to date (37 of the 43) relate broadly (and not surprisingly given that this was EBD) to the third component: patient and staff experiences. Clearly the main focus in the pilot has been on improving patient experiences. One obvious example are the changes to the physical environment of the outpatient clinic:

> *the outpatients clinic is so much better . . . It was dreadful, and a terrifying place when I first came down, and now it's much calmer, the seating's been rearranged and it's much better, and we don't have to wait two hours now before we get seen by our consultant.* (patient)

> *one thing that has improved is their feelings about the clinic . . . they are certainly saying the clinic feels better so they know what it was like and they know what it's like now. And it feels better, feels less rushed, less crowded, less threatening and so on; so that important part of their experience has changed.* (support staff)

A second example are the improvements in patient information and particularly that of the information available on the fitting, ongoing maintenance and eventual removal of the PEG feeding tube. Many of the negative feelings around this issue – bewilderment, ambiguity, fear, vulnerability – were 'designed out' as a result of these improvements:

> *One of the most important things was pre-PEG. With pre-PEG we're making sure that our information meeting and appointment times are timely. We can't change the fact that we've got to be involved at a really busy time, when they're being bombarded with information, but it's how do we best sit within that, and what appointment times do we give, so we try and give them a choice of appointments, so they feel a sense of involvement. So that was one [improvement] that happened very quickly, and the middle bit was about information, the one that really is continuing: so we've looked at pre-PEG information, information that's given at the time of the PEG insertion, so when most of the training is being given. That booklet is the biggest out of all three, and that one is the one that we've got to continue working on. The third bit of information is about when your patient is discharged, and when someone is having a PEG removed. There was a big information gap to the patients, and they were saying, 'well, I went and had my PEG removed without sedation'. So does that mean that we weren't getting it right, we weren't telling the patients, or advising them what their choices were? Why would we think that they would just have it done with a bit of local anaesthetic spray to the back of the throat?* (nursing staff)

In fact, improving information available to patients was the most common change made to improve both cognitive and emotional experiences (encompassing issues such as explaining the financial benefits available to patients, finding your way around the hospital, advice on pain management, better explanation of what radiotherapy 'planning' entailed, responding to patients' spiritual needs, a range of issues surrounding the giving and receiving of the diagnosis, and guidance as to the use and maintenance of PEG feeding tubes). Changes to physical environments (not only to the outpatient clinic but also to the post-surgical ward) were the second most common type of 'aesthetic' improvements. Less common – but no less important – were changes in staff behaviour and greater community support for patients in terms of, for example, a 'buddy' scheme.

2 What did patients and staff perceive as the central characteristics of the EBD approach?

Interviewees highlighted what were for them the four key characteristics of an EBD approach: patient involvement; patient responsibility and empowerment; a sense of community; and a close connection between their experiences and the subsequent interventions that were made in order to improve those experiences.

Patient involvement

In keeping with the philosophy underpinning the EBD approach, participants confirmed that the high levels of patient involvement throughout the whole pilot had been a key feature of the work. Participants spoke of 'more coming from the patient', 'patients identifying their own gaps and pushing forward with things they want' and 'the patients having done the work':

> *the difference between trying to make improvements in the past and this [EBD] process is that patients are involved right from the beginning. That to me is what makes the difference and that's why I feel there has been greater progress and greater improvement in the head and neck service, whereas in the past it's just fizzled out.* (support staff)

> *So actually the patients have done the work, if that makes sense. So we have worked alongside the patients, and I think to me that has been one of the most positive aspects of the whole project. We try and say we treat patients as equals when we are working alongside them and we obviously build up a very good relationship with patients from a therapy point of view. Perhaps unlike some of the consultants, we get to know them a lot better, but it is still not really collaboration or a partnership, whereas I think this was much more on an equal footing. That was really, really positive.* (therapist)

Patient responsibility

Related to the above characteristic, participants also spoke of how the EBD process had given patients a greater sense of direct responsibility for the work and its outcomes (and as one staff member pointed out, 'using patients is an efficiency in itself'!):

> *an opportunity for patients to take responsibility, because I think with this sort of treatment and experience, it's essential that the patients take some responsibility for their own well-being. What I mean by that is to bring about change, to improve the experience, not just for themselves but for others following on.* (patient)

> *It surprised me how committed they are. They are always at meetings, always on time. Their commitment has really blown me away because I know normally when you have got patient groups, sometimes you'll have four, next time you got one and then it is a bit* ad hoc *but this time they have been really committed and I would praise them for that.* (support staff)

Sense of community

Key to the success of the pilot has been the strong relationship that has grown up between patients and staff over this short period of time. This team or community aspect was remarked upon consistently by all those we interviewed:

> *There is a greater sense of community. We know the staff and I think that's bene-fited us as well . . . it's a bit like being on a train – everybody sitting there in stony silence but if the train breaks down and you're sitting there for a while together, people start to talk. It's a common sort of purpose where people bond under adver-sity. And obviously we've got to know staff a lot better and we're communicating and interacting with the staff and that becomes infectious with other people; you find that you speak to other patients that you don't know so well.* (patient)

> *for me that's been one of the biggest features; I think there has been a commu-nity. I call it a community in that staff and patients talk to each other and have these conversations, there's conversations going on in clinic, people might put stuff on the blog. People are asking, when's the next meeting? People are stand-ing at the event last week in small groups chatting to each other, they are see-ing each other much more, a group of people who are doing this work together. So for me the community bit is probably the strongest thing; the fact that these patients didn't talk to each other before, they didn't talk to staff like this before and staff didn't talk to patients like this before.* (support staff)

> *a way, actually, to build a network which includes both patients and staff and some sort of a community because initially it's obviously quite a difficult and isolated thing being a patient, sitting in the clinic, wondering what is going to be said to you, what the future is, and generally being quite apprehensive, and there are a whole lot of other people around you who are probably all feeling the same but nobody knows anybody else and it's very rare for people to have the courage to actually speak to anybody else. But there's a completely different atmosphere once there are two or three people who know each other and it is an opportunity to include others so it's important that it's not exclusive just to those who know each other because of this project.* (patient)

The connection between experiences and improvements

The fourth and final characteristic is an important one, we believe, in terms of positioning EBD in relation to other narrative-type approaches to improvement. For instance, as we discussed in Chapter 8, many of the features of a discovery interview (DI) and the discovery process itself are the same or very similar to those in the EBD process. However, the connection between story, service design and real action/improvement may still end up being quite weak or even non-existent. This, we believe, is where EBD has something very new and special to offer. As one staff member put it in the pilot of the EBD approach:

> *for me this is about 'Oh God, they're our patients aren't they?' When people watch the film they might think, 'I remember that guy', they know they're our patients – they can't get away from the fact – but it actually makes it more real for them. Whatever way they're captured, it's about capturing it so that people recog-nise these are patients I have cared for, nursed, met, who are saying this . . . and I think that's what is so different from other improvement work in terms of*

things like discovery interviews and focus groups: it's that direct connection between them.

The result of this 'connection' is, in our view, a much higher level of clinical engagement in the improvement effort than we have usually observed in other improvement projects, as suggested by the following quotation from another staff member:

and I've just found myself being more and more involved and actually you can't get away from it if you're going to work as a team, and that's what you want to do, then you can't ignore it. You're either in there or you're not in there and almost you get left behind. (nursing staff)

I never once had the impression that the clinical staff were being forced to participate in this; from the professional point of view, I never had that impression at all that it was something that was being foisted upon them, or imposed upon them; it was something that they really wanted to do. (patient)

I think it's quite moving actually. Every time I sit and attend one of these big meetings and I listen to the person talking, I feel really moved. I mean quite emotional, actually, and it's lovely when they say such positive things about everybody. (nursing staff)

Such sentiments and the sense of community that grew around the pilot (*see* earlier quotations) suggest to us a much more 'social movement'-type approach to change[30] where the improvement effort takes on a life and energy of its own. In the following section we also illustrate how these high levels of clinical involvement did not feel merely 'token' to patients but significant and substantial.

3 What did participants identify as the 'must-do's' or key success factors of an EBD approach?

Summative evaluation is very much about finding the right 'design principles' (*see* Chapter 7) for the design of future improvement processes. In essence the following are the 10 principles, prerequisites, imperatives or 'must do's' if EBD is to work as effectively as it has seemed to do in the pilot based on the views of the participants. Many of these will be familiar to any good organisational development (OD) process, and that is because EBD is very much designed as an OD process, not simply a specific tool or technique. As we have argued elsewhere,[31] the EBD approach is not some great leap forward but rather a re-conceptualisation of the OD process and aims. Our proposition is that it is within the co-analysis and co-design by staff and users (employing concepts such as 'touch points' and 'design rules') that EBD can help forge new directions for OD, whilst at the same time OD can bring change models and skills to EBD that designers in other fields may lack. These then are the 10 'must do's' from the co-designers of the EBD pilot themselves (i.e. the patients and staff who jointly led the work).

i Stay true to the core methodology especially the notion of co-design: it seems to work!

In particular, retain the following key components: patients and staff co-designing services together and on an equal footing; the use of moving/mobilising narratives and stories; connecting such narratives to improvement interventions; the use of touch points as the focus for the intervention; and a process of ongoing evaluation for learning.

ii A local improvement specialist to have dedicated time to co-ordinate the work and support frontline clinical staff

Coming up with a method that works is one thing, getting it to work, that is successful execution, is quite another. In common with many other improvement projects that have been evaluated in the NHS over the last 5 or 6 years, one key success factor is the availability of sufficient 'slack' in the system to allow staff time to actually do improvement. In the case of this pilot this 'slack' had been provided by the local service improvement facilitator who had led the work locally, and without whom, everyone agrees, the EBD project would not have succeeded.

iii Engage relevant clinical champions and senior executive support (and link the work back in to the 'normal' management processes within the organisation)

As we discuss elsewhere, people had reported that the pilot had been successful in engaging significantly high levels of clinical support, not least because of the commitment made at the outset to develop a close working relationship between researchers, nursing and management staff and senior clinicians. However, the pilot was less successful in linking the work back in to the 'normal' management processes of the organisation. For example, it was not until relatively late in the process that the actions integrated in any way back into the surgical directorate. Although individual staff members in relevant management posts were involved in the initial staff interviews and the staff feedback event, for a significant period at the beginning of the pilot there was no explicit process to ensure implementation and the work was mainly achieved through the enthusiasm and goodwill of the staff involved 'on the ground'. In part, this was due to the inevitable uncertainty around which touch points would be prioritised at the first co-design event.

iv Make use of a third party to observe and feedback on existing service(s) to staff, and forge strong links between research and practice

Many of those involved with the process were in favour of retaining the third-party research(er) component. The senior surgeon on the advisory group was concerned that an EBD process that jumped the initial research stage would not capture the key issues and challenges (or touch points) in as effective a way as the researchers had done. Other reasons for retaining this component included: patients and carers might prefer to raise and talk through issues with a non-partisan third party without staff being present, and that – through their observational role – the researchers had been able to see things that staff (and even sometimes patients) had not been aware of or able to see (certainly the weighing scales, red line and language in the consultation – crucial touch points described earlier – would not have been identified). Whilst it is recognised that not all EBD projects will have the resources for external researchers, the summative recommendation – from the comments of those involved – would be to include them if possible, recognising that it is not just about data gathering or analysis (which internal staff could learn to do for themselves over time) but the fact that the very presence of a third party will affect the dynamics of the process. For instance, significant time was invested at the beginning of the pilot in relationship and commitment building with relevant staff and patients, and some senior clinicians said that the presence and close involvement of academics had provided a further spur to their participation.

v Invest significant time with patients at the beginning of the EBD process

Some participants were also concerned that moving too quickly to the co-design group stage might result in an unequal partnership between patients and staff. The consensus was that it can only be 'co-design' if people feel equal and there is shared ownership of the process with both committed to trying to improve the patient (and staff) experience. Staff felt that the time spent at the beginning of the pilot with patients was a very good investment. One of the early challenges of the EBD process is putting patients and carers 'back in touch' with their experiences, and helping them to recall and re-live them in the here and now. This does not just happen, the initial task of this research/story-gathering phase being to trigger this reflective, retrospective 'sensemaking' process, and an attitude of wanting to re-visit the experience among the participants and share it with others.

vi Ensure that there is a range of ways in which patients can get involved by employing a number of different tools for engagement

During the pilot various methods of engaging patients and staff in the work were tested (including posters in the outpatient clinic, a project newspaper, patient diaries, staff logs, disposable cameras, and a project website). Some of these were more successful than others (the diaries, staff logs and cameras were not extensively used – and there probably was a case of overload or overkill – and some staff members also commented that they had not found the website particularly helpful) but all of these methods played a part in the branding and advertising of the project. The most effective way of recruiting patients to the work appeared to be through personal approaches from clinical staff (and in some cases this was assisted by the patients having previously read the project newspaper or seen the poster in the clinic). In part related to the concerns that some interviewees had regarding how representative the patients who took part were of the larger patient group (*see* later comments), it was felt important to offer a range of different ways in which patients could participate in an EBD process.

vii Allow patients and staff space and time to talk about their personal experiences of the service

Patients and staff alike felt that it was essential to have a way of capturing patient experiences in particular, and that time and space was needed in the overall process in order for this to happen:

> *certainly for me an interview is essential. I don't see how you can deal with an experience unless there's some foundation to it . . . I don't think you could do a project of this nature without a good in-depth interview.* (patient)

viii   Use film of patient and staff stories wherever possible

Again we recognise that it may not be possible for all future EBD projects to make extensive use of film as a way of capturing patient and staff stories and then engaging with a wider audience around the issues raised. Nevertheless, the use of film in this pilot was undoubtedly seen as one of the key success factors in the pilot. We use the term 'mobilising narratives' to describe the power of stories to move people but the same applies to 'mobilising images', if not more so:

> *I hadn't seen the film before and I thought it was good to hear from the patients what they thought, because their perceptions and our perceptions are two completely different things. I think it would be good if everybody did that. I think it is alright doing a survey on paper but a survey on paper is only as good as any patient is willing to write at the end of the day, or limited in that way, but to actually sit down and see their faces and hear their emotion, I think it is a good impact and it made you think.* (support staff)

> *I think some way of capturing experiences and being able to replay them is useful because people could revisit that or listen to it again . . . that's a huge benefit in terms of keeping the engine of motivation going, reinforcing the work and pulling people into it who couldn't be there on the day and therefore beginning to impact on people . . . it would be much harder to do that without the film.* (support staff)

ix   Maintain a high profile for the project in the organisation

The advisory group for the pilot was chaired by the Director of Nursing and its members included the General Manager responsible for Clinical Support Services (with some responsibility for cancer nursing and other teams and – at the time – also acting as Clinical Director for Pathology, Pharmacy and Therapies) and the lead clinician from the head and neck service. The chief executive of the Trust was kept updated of progress of the pilot by the local service improvement facilitator, and attended the advisory group from time to time (as well as the second co-design event with patients and staff). As a result of this, the pilot became part of the organisation's 'quality story'[8] and was highlighted by the chief executive and others in various public forums as an example of his and the organisation's commitment to improving patient experiences.

x   Plan ahead for each successive phase by recruiting new patients and carers

How can an EBD approach become embedded in the day-to-day practice of a service so that all patients have an opportunity to talk directly with staff about their experiences, and how might they work alongside staff in seeking to improve them? According to those involved, what seems to be needed are better tools to enable staff to work in a co-design way with all patients as a part of their usual jobs, thereby embedding the approach in normal behavioural routines. Alternative ways of reaching out to and engaging reticent or reluctant patients are now being considered, the key to which seems to be making the interaction as natural and 'unevent-like' as possible for them. For example, one idea adopted from IDEO in the US[32] might be to design a series of 'conversation cards' with which to initiate conversation with patients and family members. Patients in the waiting area could be invited (by staff in rotation) to look through the cards and choose a topic of most interest or concern to them in terms of the experiences they are having at that time. The cards act as an invitation to talk and help trigger a conversation between the patients and care providers around experiences and touch points, free of the burden of having to attend full-blown co-design meetings or events.

One specific suggestion from a member of staff in the pilot (not dissimilar to IDEO's above but in the consulting room rather than the waiting room) was to make questions about the patient's experience a routine part of the consultation:

> *some patients know that they don't want to join a big group and yet they have one comment . . . there should be a way . . . in terms of involving clinicians we could have a set of questions to ask so that we don't forget, so every single patient we talk to we discuss with them a certain list of non-medical items that we commit to notes . . . because to me that is true doctoring rather than a 'surgeon' or a 'radiotherapist' or what-not. That's the difference between a 'surgeon' and a 'doctor'.* (surgeon)

By using conversational analysis techniques (e.g. touch-point analysis; *see also* Chapter 8) staff could then begin to prioritise and implement their joint improvement efforts with a smaller, core group of patients but this time based on a much wider canvas of opinion across a more representative patient sample. As one patient described it, such an approach would lend itself naturally to the challenge of cultural change on which the spread and sustainability of the approach would rest or fall:

> *Of course maybe staff will also need something which will reassure them that it's okay to accept somebody's criticism or even to spend time talking to a patient because of course that's always been a thing that nurses should do but if they dare to do it, what are you doing, standing there doing nothing? It is a very big cultural change and it's probably for absolutely everybody employed in the hospital, volunteers, admitted to the hospital or visiting the hospital, from cleaners to the chief executive.* (patient)

4 What can the pilot tell us about the likely spread and sustainability of improvements brought about by an EBD approach?

The improvement specialist from the hospital, who was a vital member of the project core team and the one closest to the day-to-day EBD process, viewed the more 'general effects of the work' as being those listed on page 153, at the end of Chapter 9. The additional attraction so far as EBD is concerned seems to be, therefore, that in contrast with traditional improvement methods it appears able to achieve success on all three fronts: implementation, spread and sustainability. On the sustainability question, for example, Canny[33] has recently concluded from his review of some of the great design achievements in the last 50 years (such as the personal computer, office information systems, the internet, and mobile phone) that, 'When you execute the human-centred design process well you get a design that endures for decades'. This is the same argument that we believe can be made in relation to health service design: strive to design a service that scores high on P, E *and* A (*see* earlier) and successful spread and sustainability will be all the more likely.

Spread

As well as the planned future use of an EBD approach on other ongoing projects in the Trust, there were two specific examples of unplanned spread noted by staff (natural spread being another feature of a movement-like change dynamic within the improvement process). First, some of the changes to the physical environment of the outpatients clinic were noted by the managers of other outpatient departments in the hospital and replicated therein:

> *I definitely think it is of benefit for other services and other people who have been involved in the service, like outpatients, that they are now looking and they're taking aspects of the project and they're actually expanding it to the general outpatient area.* (nursing staff)

Second, the changes made to the policy on how much choice head and neck patients could have on when their PEG was fitted, and the information they received relating to the device, were to be made available to *all* patients requiring PEG feeding tubes:

> *with the PEGs, other groups of patients have PEGs inserted so that's another way that information is going to be incorporated for all the PEG patients, so that's another thing they're taking forward and spreading.* (nursing staff)

Sustainability

The advisory group for the pilot identified three main potential drivers for sustainability: (a) patients and carers carrying on with the work for themselves; (b) staff feeling sufficiently energised by the process and the mobilising narratives that had been heard and seen; and (c) 'old-fashioned' management systems. It is likely that all three of the above drivers would need to be active if improvements identified by an EBD process were to be first implemented and then sustained. Qualitative evidence would suggest that (a) and (b) were active in this particular pilot. Regarding the latter, one staff member commented:

> *you can see a progressive change over time in the way in which they get more confident in working with patients and can talk to them about stuff that isn't clinical; I've seen that change. I certainly know people like x and y, they think about the way in which the patients can be involved, more so now than earlier on. I can see that they seem to be envisaging a future where they will work with patients rather than without them. I can't see now that they can see themselves going backwards and not doing things at least somewhat in that way.* (support staff)

However, regarding point (c), it was not until near the end of the pilot that the core team came to realise that the EBD actions had not been integrated into the broader management responsibilities and processes of the surgical directorate. The conclusion of this evaluation is that implementation does need to occur as part of an extracurricular process (so as to allow all the special things we observed – energy, passion, momentum – to manifest and express themselves) but that sustainability and spread require the judicious use of the mainstream management system and all the skills and resources available to it. In this particular pilot we took action in this direction by firming up the list of changes that each of the six groups had signed up to; this became the core group's checklist for monitoring (against agreed deadlines) what had or had not been done by the time of the second co-design event. Members of the core team then began to meet regularly with the chief executive of the hospital to (a) ensure that the ongoing work was integrated into the wider improvement efforts of the organisation; and (b) anchor the identified priorities into the performance management systems in the hospital.

Looking to the future, staff in particular felt that in order for the improvements and work to date to be sustained, the ongoing availability of a skilled co-ordinator for the work would be key:

> *have somebody like [the service improvement facilitator], just occasionally just pulling everyone together saying where have you got to, so if people and work are falling by the wayside a bit for whatever reason, they could just sort of address those issues. So [she]'s obviously been very, very much involved but I think some of the work, in smaller groups, we can just carry on with it but I just think you need someone there just to keep an eye and make sure things don't fall by the wayside.* (nursing staff)

Both patients and staff were very aware of the need to recruit new and additional patients to sustain the forward momentum of the process. Whilst many of the individual co-design groups had continued to 'recruit' new patients and carers on an *ad hoc* basis, it was recognised that a more coherent strategy was needed, thereby broadening the experiences upon which the service as a whole can draw and so identifying and working to improve new touch points:

> *I think what we need to do is make sure that we keep inviting new people into the group, to keep this rolling forward, because hopefully they will be experiencing the changes that we're putting into place now, and can comment on that and maybe build on those, and say whether they're working or not.* (nursing staff)

One interesting development – which we would strongly recommend on the basis of our findings – has been the way in which some of the original patients involved in the pilot have begun to recruit other patients they have met during their treatment and follow-up into the work. Using the original patients in this way was seen as a good recruitment strategy.

To draw this chapter to an end we would say that part of the ethos of EBD is to learn as much as possible from experience – not just patient experience but also the experience of actually using an EBD method and approach. The experience of EBD in the pilot we have described and evaluated has been a wholly positive one and it is hoped that 'service dialogues' between staff and users, with both learning to think like each other, may ultimately become a common and enduring feature on the NHS improvement landscape. As to the form that an EBD evaluation should take, we hope that the case has been made for both formative and summative evaluation, especially of the qualitative, interview-based kind, and a note of caution sounded about the dangers of relying, as the NHS currently does, on satisfaction surveys alone.

References

1 Allen A, Reichfield FF, Hamilton B. The three 'D's of customer experience. *Harvard Management Update*. 2005; 7 November.

2 Fisher B. *Patients as Teachers – 'What Works For You?' A New Way of Involving Users in Improving Services*. Unpublished paper on two 'patients as teachers' initiatives in Lambeth, Southwark and Lewisham Health Authority; 2005.

3 Bate SP, Robert G. Studying health care 'quality' qualitatively: the dilemmas and tensions between different forms of evaluation research within the UK National Health Service. *Qualitative Health Research*. 2002; **12**(7): 966–81.

4 Bate SP, Robert G. Where next for policy evaluation? Insights from researching NHS Modernisation. *Policy and Politics*. 2003; **31**(2): 237–51.

5 Ling T. Ex ante evaluation and the changing public audit function. The scenario planning approach. *Evaluation*. 2003; **9**(4): 437–52.

6 Alexander H. Health service evaluations: should we expect the results to change practice? *Evaluation*. 2003; **9**(4): 405–14.

7 Dart J, Davies R. A dialogical, story-based evaluation tool: the most significant change technique. *American Journal of Evaluation*. 2003; **24**(2): 137–51.

8 Marnane K, Price C, Schaninger B. *Dialogue-Based Planning*. London: McKinsey & Company; 2005.

9 The Improvement Network, East Midlands. The Patient Centreometer. *See:* www.tin.nhs.uk/ index.asp?pgid=912 (accessed 18 September 2006).

10 Pettersen KI, Veensrtra M, Guldvog B *et al.* The patient experiences questionnaire: development, validity and reliability. *International Journal of Quality in Health Care*. 2004; **16**: 453–63.

11 Garratt AM, Bjærtnes ?, Krogstad U *et al.* The OutPatient experiences questionnaire (OPEQ): data quality, reliability, and validity in patients attending 52 Norwegian hospitals. *Quality and Safety in Health Care*. 2005; **14**: 433–7.

12 Picker Institute Europe. Inpatient questionnaire. National Patient Survey, version 10. *See*: www.nhssurveys.org/docs/Inpatient_2005_core_questionnaire_v10.pdf (accessed 18 September 2006).

13 Department of Health. *Tackling Cancer: Improving the Patient Journey*. London: TSO; 2005.

14 Safran DG, Karp M, Coltin K *et al.* Measuring patients' experiences with individual primary care physicians. Results of a statewide demonstration project. *J Gen Intern Med*. 2006; **21**: 13–21.

15 Pearse J. Review of patient satisfaction measures and experience surveys for public hospitals in Australia. *See:* www.pc.gov.au/gsp/reports/consultancy/patientsatisfaction/index.html (accessed 5 September 2006).

16 Healthcare Commission. *State of Healthcare*. London: Healthcare Commission; 2005.

17 Kale S. Bright ideas. Measuring customer experience. 26 January 2005. *See:* www.urbino.net/bright.cfm?specificBright=Measuring%20Customer%20Experience (accessed 3 July 2006).

18 Sandoval GA, Brown AD, Sullivan T *et al.* Factors that influence cancer patients' overall perceptions of the quality of care. *Int J for Q in H Care*. 2006; **18**(4): 266–74.

19 Davies E, Cleary PD. Hearing the patient's voice? Factors affecting the use of patient survey data in quality improvement. *Quality and Safety in Health Care*. 2005; **14**: 428–32.

20 Rubinoff R. How to quantify the user experience. 2004. *See:* www.sitepoint.com/article/ quantify-user-experience (accessed 19 March 2006).

21 Gomoll K, Story E. *Discovering User Needs: Field Techniques You Can Use*. Milwaukee, WI: Gomoll Research & Design; 2003. *See:* http://sigchi.org/chi2003/docs/t11.pdf (accessed 3 August 2006).

22 Jesson J. Mystery shopping demystified: is it a justifiable research method? *The Pharmaceutical Journal*. 2004; **272**: 615–17.

23 News release. Researchers at MSU, Publicom identify seven dimensions of customer experience. *See:* http://newsroom.msu.edu/site/indexer/2612/content.htm (accessed 18 September 2006).

24 Department of Health. *Autumn Performance Report 2004*. London: The Stationery Office; 2004.

25 Healthcare Commission website. *See:* www.healthcarecommission.org.uk/ nationalfindings/surveys/patientsurveys.cfm (accessed 18 September 2006).

26 Department of Health. *Autumn Performance Report 2005*. London: The Stationery Office; 2005.

27 Healthcare Commission press release. Healthcare watchdog publishes views of patients at all NHS acute hospitals. 26 May 2006. *See:* www.healthcarecommission.org.uk// newsandevents/pressreleases.cfm?cit_id=3855&FAArea1=customWidgets.content_ view_1&usecache=false (accessed 18 September 2006).

28 Coulter A. Can patients assess the quality of health care? Patients' surveys should ask about the real experiences of medical care. *British Medical Journal*. 2006; **333**: 1–2.

29 Rao M, Clarke A, Sanderson C *et al*. Patients' own assessments of quality of primary care compared with objective records based measures of technical quality of care: cross sectional study. *British Medical Journal*. 2006; **333**: 19–22.

30 Bate SP, Robert G, Bevan H. The next phase of health care improvement: what can we learn from social movements? *Quality and Safety in Health Care*. 2004; **13**(1): 62–6.

31 Bate SP, Robert G. Towards more user-centric organisational development: lessons from a case study of experience-based design. *Journal of Applied Behavioral Science*. 2007; **43**(1): 41–66.

32 Coughlan P, Fulton Suri J, Canales K. Prototypes as (design) tools for behavioral and organizational change: a design-based approach to help organizations change work behaviors. *Journal of Applied Behavioral Science*. 2007; **43**(1): 122–34.

33 Canny J. The future of human-computer interaction. *Human Computer Interaction*. 2006; **4**(6): 1–4.

Chapter 11

Future directions for experience-based design and user-centred improvement and innovation

> *We have artists with no scientific knowledge and scientists with no artistic knowledge and both with no spiritual sense of gravity at all, and the result is not just bad, it is ghastly. The time for real reunification of art and technology is really long overdue.* (Robert Pirsig)

To date, the involvement of users in co-designing services and experiences has been less prevalent in healthcare than has been the case in the field of design and in the many organisations with whom the design professionals have been working. Here there has been a proliferation of approaches, models, tools and techniques for capturing and incorporating knowledge from users' past experiences of a product or service into design processes for future products and services. In this sense there is undoubtedly some catching up to be done, and it is our hope that this book will have proved sufficient for healthcare improvement professionals, and of course patients and carers, to want to interest themselves in doing that.

It is not simply a case of following, however. There are wider developments of which even the design professions themselves currently seem only vaguely aware, which, if combined with the kind of EBD practices that have been described, could provide something groundbreaking in terms of where the NHS now finds itself and where it might be. For these we need to look not in the field of design, but innovation, which takes us to our final chapter and some speculations on what the future might hold for EBD, and in what direction it may be able to take healthcare improvement, even to the point where it may lead rather than follow.

In this, the final, chapter, we discuss three wider organisational and social trends that may not only explain the warm reception EBD has received so far, but that favour further movement by healthcare organisations in this direction in future, providing it with a highly favourable 'receptive context', and the energy to be able to progress and spread. These three trends, which point to an idea whose time has come, are:

- the trend towards democratic, user-centred innovation
- the trend towards direct user involvement in designing their own experiences
- the trend towards innovating user communities.

The trend towards democratic, user-centred innovation and improvement

Innovation and improvement should go together: an innovation should be an improvement on an existing design (innovation being the means to improvement), otherwise what is the point (recall our square lavatory seat from earlier)? But frequently they do not. This has certainly been the case in UK public services, where service design and improvement professionals have rarely turned to the innovation field for inspiration, while at the same time people working on innovation in service delivery, including ourselves,[1] have shown little interest in improvement innovations *per se*. Conceptually, the fields have been far apart, and remain so. This is somewhat different from what one might find in US and Canadian public services, where in the case of bodies like the Office of Innovation and Improvement, the concepts have become more closely intertwined.

All this now looks set to change. The NHS Modernisation Agency, which also never made any explicit connection between innovation and improvement in the past (preferring instead to focus almost exclusively on the latter), was replaced in July 2005 by the NHS Institute for Innovation and Improvement, whose title says it all in terms of the new dual focus. Its all-embracing purpose was set out in a document[2] that stated that:

> The NHS Institute will work at national level to integrate, promote and support innovation, learning, leadership and improvement in the NHS.

For the first time in the NHS innovation and improvement have therefore been deliberately and explicitly brought together. So what relevance does this have to design and especially the role of users in service design? We believe the answer may be found inside the covers of a recent seminal book on innovation called *Democratising Innovation* by MIT Professor Eric von Hippel.[3] In it, Von Hippel draws attention to the growing role of users in innovation processes – what he terms 'democratised, user-centred innovation systems' – and the associated phenomenon of the 'innovating user'. What this development requires from all of us now, he argues, is a re-conceptualisation of innovation, and of whom and what an innovation process will involve in future. A recent review of this book by Virginia Postrel of the *New York Times* summarises von Hippel's new vision of future innovation processes, pointing out that it is to some extent already with us:

> When most people think about where new or improved products come from, they imagine two kinds of innovators: either engineers and marketers in big companies trying to 'find a need and fill it' or garage entrepreneurs hoping to strike it rich by inventing the next big thing.[4]

But a lot of significant innovations today do not come from people like these trying to figure out what customers may want. They come from the users themselves, who know exactly what they want but cannot get it in existing products.

> A growing body of empirical work shows that users are the first to develop many, and perhaps most, new industrial and consumer products.[3]

The observation that 'many, and perhaps most' of today's innovations are coming from users themselves will come as a surprise to many, especially if it is true, as von Hippel claims, that this applies to service as well as product innovation. The trend towards user-led innovation, says the author, is already evident, representing a major departure from tradition, and bringing with it new and radically different kinds of processes, practices, and above all, opportunities:

> The idea that novel products and services are developed by manufacturers is deeply ingrained in both traditional expectations and scholarship. When we as

users of products complain about the shortcomings of an existing product or wish for a new one, we commonly think that 'they' should develop it – not us. Even the conventional term for an individual end user, 'consumer,' implicitly suggests that users are not active in product and service development. Nonetheless, there is now very strong empirical evidence that product development and modification by both user firms and users as individual consumers is frequent, pervasive, and important.[3]

Evidence gathered for his book led the author to conclude that:

- users' abilities to develop high-quality new products and services for themselves are improving radically and rapidly
- users develop and modify products and services for themselves and often freely reveal what they have done
- often users can be interested in adopting the solutions that other 'lead users' have developed.

It has apparently been the bigger trend toward an open and distributed innovation process driven by steadily better and cheaper computing and communications that has enabled all this to happen, and now to accelerate. This is where von Hippel's book converges and joins forces with another recent bestseller, Tom Friedman's *The World is Flat*[5] – 'flat' (which might also be read as 'connected') referring to new open-sourcing electronic technologies which allow innovations to spread easily, rapidly and cheaply across boundaries and to anywhere in the world, including user-created innovations which no longer require a corporate development context or diffusion mechanism but can easily be spread by a single person via laptop computer and the internet.

User innovation is not new, of course; in fact it has been around since the dawn of time (for example, machines and machine tools were invented by 'common workmen', driven by the need to solve a problem or accomplish a task). However, it is the scale and speed of this that makes it different today. Von Hippel gives many examples of this innovation phenomenon, one being acrobatic kitesurfing which was initially developed by an informal group of user-enthusiasts taking part in the Hawaiian surfing championships (what he terms an 'innovation niche') but which ultimately spread worldwide, giving rise to a booming industry in high-performance windsurfing kite boards with global sales of more than $100 million in 2003.

Readers will have noticed that 'user-centred innovation' is, of course, none other than our own 'user-centred design', and if this is aimed at improving the user experience, which it usually is, then this also makes it 'experience-based design' (EBD). The design process itself is also identical, almost always beginning with the need to 'scratch a personal itch': the surfer longs for more excitement and adventure than he or she is getting just riding the waves (i.e. a novel or more satisfying or fulfilling experience). Wouldn't it be great if we could fly as well as surf? But how? Begin by fitting some crude toe-traps to the board, so that you stay with the board when you take off and it does not come crashing down on your head. Modify it, tinker with it, keep on improving it until you get it right (prototyping and pilot testing), and the experience gets better and better.

One major surprise to the author and his colleagues as they began to look at highly lucrative areas such as open-source software was how willing people were to share their design freely and free of charge with each other ('free revealing'), even when it had already involved them in a lot of private expense or, by giving it away, could lead to the loss of potentially great personal wealth. Apparently, the reason is that the creation process is so addictive and intrinsically satisfying that it becomes an end in itself, plus the fact that your innovation is such a source of personal pride that you want to go out and share it with others.

This may also explain why EBD, as a form of innovation and improvement, possesses similar qualities of free revealing and free giving (just look at the amount people were prepared to give freely, willingly and voluntarily to the EBD process described in Chapter 9). For exactly the same reasons, we believe, people are drawn to a process that is sociable and interactive, novel, creative and stretching, and they want to come together to work in a highly creative context, on something they believe is worth doing, and that will ultimately be an improvement for someone's 'life experience' – a someone not unlike them, in a situation in which they may be, or may already have found themselves. This is why they give their time so freely and voluntarily, why the improvement/innovation process possesses such internal energy and drive, and why it mostly manages and takes care of itself, seemingly not requiring an organisational context or resources to continue and carry on. It is the creativity and valency of the task and process that has these powerful motivational effects, liberating what often seems to be a boundless generosity and energy. This is the kind of 'generative' innovation and improvement that does not need external levers or drivers; the drive comes from the inside, or as we have found ourselves saying on many occasions, 'You don't need an engine when you have wind in the sails.'

Continuing a little further with von Hippel's work, all design processes work the same way, says the author (*see* Figure 11.1).

Take the creation of the skateboard as a rather way-out example. In phase 1 of the cycle, the user combines need and solution information into a product idea: 'I am bored with roller skating. How can I get down this hill in a more exciting way? Maybe it would be fun to put my skates' wheels under a board and ride down on that.' In phase 2, the user builds a prototype by taking his skates apart and hammering the wheels onto the underside of a board. In phase 3, he runs the experiment by climbing onto the board and heading down the hill. In phase 4, he picks himself up from an inaugural crash and thinks about the error information he has gained: 'It is harder to stay on this thing than I thought. What went wrong, and how can I improve things before my next run down the hill?'[3]

This is exactly the kind of design process we have been describing in this book, with staff and user involved in every step of that process. This is the ultimate in user design and one that is predicated on the assumption that people will be motivated to do this willingly. On this, von Hippel says there is no doubt:

> *Individual users can sometimes be more inclined to innovate than one might expect because they sometimes value the process of innovation as well as the novel product or service that is created.*[3]

So the advantages of user-based innovation, like EBD, are clear: people want to do it, and they are prepared to do it for free. (Cynics might say this is self-exploitation but the same could be said of someone working in a charity shop or giving up their Saturday mornings in order to coach the local children's football team; the issue is one of free choice.) The other advantage is that it has the potential to

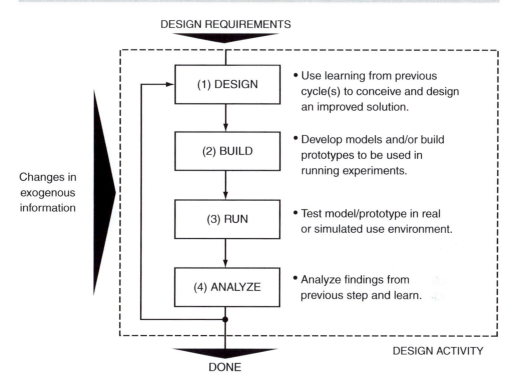

Figure 11.1   The trial-and-error cycle of product development. *Source:* von Hippel.[3] Reproduced with permission of The MIT Press.

produce a better design than even the experts or formal design departments are able to come up with because it can directly tap into the knowledge and experience of 'lead users', people at the front edge of a product or service (and who could be more lead user than a current or recently treated patient?), and who are ahead of the majority, designing things today that the majority will want tomorrow. Von Hippel is convinced that such knowledge and experience is worth a hundred expert design departments; indeed he argues that the role of these departments should not be to do the design themselves but to go out and identify and enrol lead users who will do it for them (prompting us to think first how dare they, but second who might the lead users in healthcare be?). Perhaps the 'co' in co-design will ensure that it is 'with' and not 'for' them, the notion of a partnership of equals being important to retain. However, details apart, there seems little doubt that the importance of the internal improvement process and internal improvement professionals will decline, or at least be less central, as the process opens up, this being helped along by that other trend towards more community-based participation (*see* earlier; for example, the involvement of NHS Foundation Trust members in improvement). For the NHS at least, this also represents a significant mindset change from feeling that 'they', the internal staff, should be doing the service design and development for or on behalf of the patient, to a recognition of the need for a more active, engaged patient – service development that is no longer a purely internal matter.

Another advantage of user-based design is that it is more responsive to the heterogeneity of user needs than traditional methods of design and innovation. The example von Hippel uses to illustrate this point is the mountain bike. All kinds of people go mountain biking – lawyers, company executives, families, and so on – and all have different needs and wants of the bike. Again, the advantage is that by engaging these people in the design, the product or service can be tailor-made or personalised to serve a wide range of needs and requirements. (*See* the earlier discussion in Chapter 8 about the importance of prototyping and personas in design and the kinds of method that can be brought into service to do this.)

The whole thrust of von Hippel's vision of the democratisation of innovation is that EBD, and similar user-centric innovation/improvement processes, is an idea whose time has most definitely come, and, as we said in the opening chapter, must not be allowed to simply pass healthcare by. Fortunately we do not believe this is likely to happen, with the new NHS Institute well placed to play a key role in channelling and applying these new ideas to the design of health service innovation and improvement processes.

The trend towards consumers designing their own experiences

All the way through this book we have drawn attention to the fact that EBD is made up of two elements: the first, the participation of the user in the design process, and the second, its special focus on designing experiences. We feel the case has been made for the first in our discussion of von Hippel's work, but need to show how the experience focus is also part of a wider trend and, like its partners, not an ephemeral management fad or fashion. Here we turn to another seminal piece of work, again in the innovation not improvement field, by Prahalad and Ramaswamy, aptly called 'The new frontier of experience innovation'.[6] All organisations today, the authors argue, are under pressure to create value, which in the context of healthcare obviously means value for the taxpayer, staff, and above all the patient; and value creation, they add, can only come from innovation. So how do we innovate in a way that will ensure value creation? Here we come to the authors' central argument that because of customers' increasing role in the networked society:

> *Managers are discovering that neither value nor innovation can any longer be successfully and sustainably generated through a company-centric, product-and-service-focused prism. A new point of view is required, one that allows individual customers to actively co-construct their own consumption experiences through personalised interaction, thereby co-creating unique value for themselves.*[6]

The authors have clearly retained von Hippel's user-centric emphasis but the key phrase here is 'co-construct their own consumption experiences', a phrase that takes us back to the whole point of EBD, as opposed to, say, participatory design alone. Like von Hippel, they are saying that 'experience innovation' is also a wider emerging trend in organisations and society generally, although probably less well advanced than the participatory element. This is why they are at pains to point out that we are not talking about current practices or even best practices, but next practices.

What they are sure about is that many organisations have already started transitioning from a 'product or service focus' to a 'solutions' focus, a shift that will

	Traditional Innovation	Experience Innovation
Focus of Innovation	Products and processes	Experience environments
Basis of Value	Products and services	Co-creation experiences
View of Value Creation	Firm creates value	Value is co-created
	Supply-chain-centric fulfillment of products and services	Experience environments for individuals to co-construct experiences on contextual demand
	Supply push and demand pull for firm's offerings	Individual-centric co-creation of value
View of Technology	Facilitator of features and functions	Facilitator of experiences
	Technology and systems integration	Experience integration
Focus of Supply Chains	Supports fulfillment of products and services	Experience network supports co-construction of personalized experiences

Figure 11.2   Traditional innovation and experience innovation. *Source:* Prahalad and Ramaswamy.[6] Reproduced with permission of *MIT Sloan Management Review.*

only be complete when they have reached the final stage: an 'experience' focus (*see* Figure 11.2).

EBD work of the kind we have been carrying out fits – encouragingly – with this wider trend, suggesting again that the NHS may be heading in the right direction, even anticipating the trend by being able to claim it is (albeit small-scale) current practice not just next practice. Clearly, in terms of ambition, EBD has many of the characteristics of the right-hand column of Figure 11.2. On the other hand, in practice it may still be some way off this. For example, we still use the phrase 'service improvement' (EBD as a method of service improvement), which, as the authors point out, remains firmly inside the traditional paradigm, and which will only really change when we drop the phrase 'service improvement' entirely and talk directly about 'experience improvement' instead:

> *The intent of experience innovation is not to improve a product or service, per se, but to enable the co-creation of an environment populated by organisations and consumers and their networks – in which personalised, evolvable experiences are the goal, and products and services evolve as a means to that end.*[6]

Nevertheless, the early signs are promising, and it is again encouraging that EBD in healthcare will be able to pick up some of the energy from this wider social and organisational trend towards an experience focus, as it can also do with the trend towards co-creation and user-led innovation.

The trend towards innovating communities and its implication for 'spread'

There are also important links to be made here with another body of work in which we have been involved in the area of social movements and mobilisation.[7] The distinctive feature of movements is that change is faster, larger and deeper than what is normally found in organisational change programmes – a particular attraction to organisations like the NHS that are trying to bring about a 'quality revolution and a step change in results' but finding that change is slower and more incremental than desired. In regard to this issue of the scale and pace of change, we have heard how democratised user-based innovations and improvements spread rapidly to huge numbers of people, and therefore display genuine 'movement-like' tendencies (what movements theorists refer to as collective effervescence or collective contagion). Perhaps, then, user-based innovation of the EBD variety might hold an important key to 'spread' that has so far eluded healthcare improvement professionals. For example, von Hippel and colleagues found that users who freely reveal what they have done often find that others then improve or suggest improvements to the innovation to mutual benefit, effectively creating an 'improvement spiral' (which, of course, is another word for spread).

Another literature which has clear but as yet unconnected links with von Hippel and the user-innovation writers, and great relevance to both the spread and sustainability issues, has begun to develop the notion of 'innovation communities' or 'innovative communities'.[8–10] This multidisciplinary field is producing evidence to show that user-innovation communities (self-organising collaborative communities of users of the kind described by both von Hippel and Friedman) can speed up as well as improve the quality of innovation and, by the same token, improvement (www.wikipedia.org, the online encyclopaedia written by users, being a good example). The NHS has a long tradition of such collaborative communities, and it is not difficult to see how new websites such as www.dipex.org might be developed further, progressing beyond information sharing to genuine community-based innovation. The new regional NHS Innovation Hubs might also have a key role to play in this area in this regard.

More broadly than healthcare service provision, we have also recently seen the growth and spread of 'embodied health movements' (EHMs) that address disease, disability or illness experience via patients and carers challenging science on aetiology, diagnosis, treatment and prevention:[11]

> EHMs include 'contested illnesses' that are either unexplained by current medical knowledge or have environmental explanations that are disputed . . . the formation of a politicised collective illness identity that arises both out of the intersubjective experience of suffering as well as the shared political positions of marginality that come with being diagnosed with a poorly understood or characterised condition. What is key about the embodied nature of this movement, however, is that activists frame their organising efforts and critique of the system through a personal awareness and understanding of their experience. We view EHMs as organised efforts to challenge knowledge and practice concerning the aetiology, treatment, and prevention of disease. This arises from the recent trend towards the empowerment of patients and more active involvement in their health care.

EBD – the subject of this book – is but one small seed in this wider social and organisational terrain, but there is no doubt that it provides highly fertile ground for it to grow if there are enough people to tend and husband it.

A last brief word

We hope this book has gone some way towards achieving the four objectives we set for it in our opening chapter, these being:

1   to examine healthcare quality and service improvement challenges from the fresh angle of contemporary design and the service design professions, a process which will involve the exploration of new concepts, methods, and practices, most of which are currently outside the health field

2   to draw the attention of improvement researchers and practitioners in particular to the multidisciplinary field of interactive or 'user-centric' design and the whole concept of 'co-designing for user experience'
3   to take the concepts of user involvement and user experience and make them the focus of a different, and more intense, kind of attention in order to discover ways of *seeing deeper into experience*, of appreciating why it is important to be 'designing experiences' and not just systems or processes, and
4   to interest and equip readers with sufficient information, interest and understanding to go out and get involved in the 'doing' of EBD.

We have seen how the traditional view of the user as a passive recipient of a product or service has begun to give way to the new view of 'active' users as the co-designers of that product or service, integral to the improvement and innovation process. This is not to suggest that a focus on 'experience' is a panacea for all the ills in healthcare systems, for:

> *We are humans, and humans err. Despite outrage, despite grief, despite experience, despite our best efforts, despite our deepest wishes, we are born fallible and will remain so . . . Being careful helps, but it brings us nowhere near perfection . . . just 'trying harder' makes no one superhuman. Exhortation does not help much, nor will suspending the doctors, nor will outrage in the headlines, nor even will guilt.* (Donald Berwick, Institute for Healthcare Improvement, as cited in Petit-Zeman[12])

Nonetheless, even for the honest grapplers the world is becoming 'flatter', more open, more user-driven, and there is no reason to suppose that healthcare is, or should be, any different. Tom Friedman, the man who came up with the concept, has told us there is a need to stop here and take stock, and we believe this applies as much to innovation and improvement in healthcare as it does anywhere else. EBD and user-based innovation are two of the most powerful 'flattening' forces in this emerging scenario, and it is to be hoped that healthcare organisations will seek to explore and reap the benefits from them in the years to come. The message is clear: user experience has to become a core competency within the NHS, just as it is within a number of today's leading organisations.[13] There are so many reasons why this should be so: ethical, governance and safety, efficiency and performance (P, E, and A) but above all for the patient and carer experience itself which must surely hold the key to restoration of the 'noble idea' in healthcare.

References

1   Greenhalgh T, Robert G, Bate SP *et al. Diffusion of Innovations in Health Service Organisations.* Oxford: Blackwell; 2005.
2   Department of Health. *The Way Forward. The NHS Institute for Learning, Skills and Innovation.* London: The Stationery Office, 2005.
3   Von Hippel E. *Democratising Innovation.* Cambridge, MA: The MIT Press; 2005.
4   Postrel V. Innovation moves from the laboratory to the bike trail and the kitchen. *New York Times.* 2005; 21 April.
5   Friedman TL. *The World is Flat: A Brief History of the 21st Century.* New York: Farrar, Straus & Giroux; 2005.
6   Prahalad CK, Ramaswamy V. The new frontier of experience innovation. *MIT Sloan Management Review.* 2003; **44**(4): 9–18.

7 Bate SP, Robert G, Bevan H. The next phase of health care improvement: what can we learn from social movements? *Quality and Safety in Health Care*. 2004; **13**(1): 62–6.

8 What indeed is a community? www.gdrc.org/sustdev/inn-comm/cs-4.html (accessed 18 September 2006).

9 Sustainable Communities Network. About sustainable communities. www.sustainable. org/information/aboutsuscom.html (accessed 18 September 2006).

10 Global Environment Information Centre. Environment area project. Innovative communities. http://geic.hq.unu.edu/env/project1.cfm?type=1&ID=255 (accessed 18 September 2006).

11 Brown P, Zavestoski S, McCormick S *et al*. Embodied health movements: new approaches to social movements in health. *Sociology of Health and Illness*. 2004; **26**(1): 50–80.

12 Petit-Zeman S. *Doctor, What's Wrong? Making the NHS Human Again*. Abingdon: Routledge; 2005.

13 Gabriel-Petit P. Why UX should matter to software companies. UXMatters.com. 2006; March.

Patient interview schedule

Note: this guide is for interviewers. A shorter version with the introduction, headings and numbered points only is sent to patients to think about in advance.

The story of your journey

Introduction

To help us to improve healthcare services for you – and for patients who have a similar illness to you – we would like you to tell us your story of your illness and treatment in your own words.

- Your confidentiality is completely assured.
- We would like to tape-record our conversation so that we can later write down all your own words to help improve services; we will not let anyone else listen to the tape without your prior permission.
- Telling us your story – or deciding not to take part – will have absolutely no effect on the treatment and care which you will receive.
- Anything too painful or distressing, tell us and we will stop.
- It will probably take about an hour but just let us know if and when you want to take a break or to stop completely.
- Or would prefer to deal with our conversation in a different way.
- We would also like to hear from anybody else who has been on the journey with you who would like to tell us about what happened – partner, relative, friend, etc. – either with you here or some other time on their own.
- If you can try and be as specific as you can about what happened and how you felt, and we are particularly keen to hear about any particular events or experiences, good or bad.

We would prefer you to tell us your story in your own words with as few interruptions from us as possible, but we have some prompts if you would prefer that . . .

So . . . let's begin at the beginning. Tell us your story in your own words . . .

1 Your journey so far (referral – tests and investigations – diagnosis – treatment – discharge – follow-up)

1.1 The first time you noticed something was not right

When did this all start?

  Your first reaction? Can you remember how it felt?

  Did you discuss with others? Who? What did they say?

  How long before you contacted your doctor or a healthcare professional?

  Did you try to find out any information about your illness – a medical dictionary, the internet? Talk to other people?

  What did you find out? How did the information make you feel?

What recommendations would you make to other patients about what to do in this first period?

1.2   The first meeting with your GP

What happened and what sticks in your mind about that?

What was said?

How knowledgeable/interested/concerned was he/she about your symptoms and possible diagnosis?

Although it may have been distressing, would you call it a 'good experience'?

Any ways it could have been improved?

1.3   Later meetings with GP and others in primary care

As above.

1.4   Your first trip to the hospital outpatients clinic

How long was it between seeing your GP and going to the hospital? What was it like during the gap? (worrying time? anxious?)

First impressions of the hospital and the clinic (clinic reception desk, waiting area, the general place, other people there, staff)? Good or not?

1.5   The first meeting with your consultant

Memories of that first visit?

Feelings about several people being in the room? (too many? comfort blanket?) Did you know who everyone was? Did it matter?

Did you leave feeling you knew exactly:

(a)   what was wrong with you
(b)   what your treatment options were, and
(c)   what tests you would need to have and what treatment would be involved (including side effects)? (Any issues about medical jargon, difficult words, lack of clarity, talking pace?)

Were you given too much/too little information?

Did you find it difficult to take in information at this emotional time? Were you able to take it all in?

Looking back on it now is there anything that would have helped make this initial experience better/easier? (More space/time to take it in, ask questions, clarify, pencil and paper!) What are the 'must do's', you would tell other patients to follow in that kind of situation?)

1.6   First meeting with other staff, including tests
(list – similar questions for each)

How easy was it to make the appointments and arrangements for the tests you had to have after you had seen the consultant? Was it easy to find your way around the hospital when you left the clinic?

Who else do you remember speaking to on that first visit to the hospital? Did they help? (Clinical nurse specialist, speech and language therapist, nutritionist, etc.) How did they help?

How important were other non-clinical staff during this time (receptionist, dental nurse)?

1.7 Back to family and friends

Role played by family and friends before you went in for your operation. Their response? Problematic? Supportive?

Did you meet up with any other patients with a similar illness to your own? How helpful was that? In what ways?

1.8 Treatment begins

Did you have anything else by way of care or treatment before your operation? Were there other things that had to be done before your operation? What did that involve?

Did you feel adequately prepared for what you would experience when you woke up after your surgery (discomfort, etc.)? Did you know what to expect?

Experience of your time on the ward. What sticks in your mind? Good things and bad things, things that could be better or improved on?

How long were you in hospital for after your operation? Did you feel ready to go home when you did?

Did you go to other hospitals for treatment (e.g. for radiotherapy)? What were they like? Easy to get to? What happened when you were there?

1.9 Follow-up

How much information did your GP have about what had happened to you when you went back? Was he/she well informed?

What was the nature of the follow-up support? Was it good? Where might it be improved?

Who provided that support? District nurse? Health visitor? Nutrition support? Speech and language therapist? Who did you have lots of contact with after you had gone home? Who has been the most helpful?

2 Issues

Some other questions about your experience.

Overall satisfaction

Broadly speaking, how satisfied have you been so far with the care and treatment you have received?

How does it compare with other departments or hospitals you may have been to?

Best bits and worst bits of the H & N service?

The information you received

Did you find it difficult or awkward to communicate with the medical staff?

What types of issues did you ask questions about? (Type and stage of cancer, alternative treatments and outcomes, details of the timings and process, effects on diet, lifestyle and relationships, side effects, etc.) What would you have liked more information about?

Were you clear on what was wrong and the various treatment options available to you?

Were you told or made aware of the cancer information suite on the first floor of the hospital? Did you go there?

Did you receive any written information about your diagnosis, and how easy to understand did you find it?

Did you contact BACUP or any other body for more information?

Were you given good advice as to how to find more information about your condition?

Did you always leave a meeting with your doctors knowing what was happening next?

Were there particular parts of your care and treatment where you could have done with more/less/better information?

Have there been times when you have been given conflicting or contradictory information?

Information about your treatment: were you clear about how well your treatment was progressing/how successful it had been?

Is the problem too much or too little information?

Do people in situations like yours want all the information, bad news as well as good news? Do they prefer not to know?

How much influence you had

Have you had any influence in the choice of hospital, consultant, and treatment options?

Are there any things in which you would liked to have had more 'say'?

On a scale from letting the surgeon decide what to do, to you both deciding together, to him advising you but leaving the final decision to you, which happened and which would you prefer?

We hear a lot about patient-centred care. How far have you felt at the centre of things throughout your treatment?

Your relationships with the medical staff you met

How would you describe your relationship with . . . (consultant, etc. – see list)? (Openness, trust, respect, closeness/personal, approachability, expertise, equality.) So is it paternalistic or collegial, distant or close?

So how has that relationship developed?

Are there any things that prevented or deterred you from raising issues with the medical staff?

Any problem relationships or difficult or stressful encounters with staff or others?

How far would you say you have been treated with respect, courtesy and sensitivity?

Do you feel as though staff have accompanied you on this journey, or do you feel you have done it very much on your own?

What other types of support did you have?

Professional: Can we check what local support groups outside the hospital have been helping you? (For each + stories): to what extent have they been able to play a positive role in helping you deal with the experience? (Community, belongingness/acceptance, information, practical help.) Any downsides?

Partner, family, friends, fellow workers, peers, etc. (as above).

Fellow patients (as above and on the ward/waiting room? friendships?).

Might it have/did it help to have met with previous patients?

How did you manage to cope?

What other effects has all this had on you and your health (depression, behaviour change, etc.)?

What advice would you give to other people about how to develop a personal coping strategy and how to stay in control of your own life?

3 Best and worst bits

Where would you say are the crucial points in the journey – moments of truth? Crucial touch points? The parts we should focus on in the design process? What were the best and worst parts of your whole experience?

Based on your first-hand experience, if you were looking to redesign and improve the services for H & N patients where would you begin? Imagine we were setting it all up from scratch (includes physical environment, the process itself, staff attitudes and behaviour, etc.)?

THANK YOU VERY MUCH FOR ALL YOUR HELP!

Index